MORE THAN JUST A PRETTY FACE

BY THOMAS D. REES, M.D.

Aesthetic Plastic Surgery

Cosmetic Facial Surgery

BY SYLVIA SIMMONS

How to Be the Life of the Podium

The Great Garage Sale Book

New Speakers Handbook

Dr. Neumann's Guide to the New Sexually Transmitted Diseases (with Hans H. Neumann, M.D.)

The Straight Story on V.D. (with Hans H. Neumann, M.D.)

MORE THAN JUST A PRETTY FACE

HOW COSMETIC SURGERY CAN IMPROVE YOUR LOOKS AND YOUR LIFE

THOMAS D. REES, M.D.
with SYLVIA SIMMONS

Illustrated by Leon Tadrick

LITTLE, BROWN AND COMPANY   Boston   Toronto

COPYRIGHT © 1987 BY THOMAS D. REES, M.D.,
AND SYLVIA SIMMONS

ALL RIGHTS RESERVED. NO PART OF THIS BOOK MAY BE REPRODUCED IN ANY FORM OR BY ANY ELECTRONIC OR MECHANICAL MEANS, INCLUDING INFORMATION STORAGE AND RETRIEVAL SYSTEMS, WITHOUT PERMISSION IN WRITING FROM THE PUBLISHER, EXCEPT BY A REVIEWER WHO MAY QUOTE BRIEF PASSAGES IN A REVIEW.

FIRST EDITION

In this book I tell the stories of some of my patients. To protect their privacy, all their names have been changed.

Thomas D. Rees, M.D.

Library of Congress Cataloging-in-Publication Data
Rees, Thomas D.
  More than just a pretty face.
  1. Face — Surgery. 2. Surgery, Plastic.
I. Simmons, S. H. (Sylvia H.) II. Title. [DNLM:
1. Face — surgery — popular works. 2. Surgery, Plastic — popular works. WE 705 R328m]
RD119.5.F33R44   1987   617'.520592   86-27617
ISBN 0-316-73707-0

RRD VA

Designed by Patricia Girvin Dunbar

*Published simultaneously in Canada
by Little, Brown & Company (Canada) Limited*

PRINTED IN THE UNITED STATES OF AMERICA

For
NAN

Contents

1 Improving One's Looks: A Universal Desire   3
2 Cosmetic Surgery Comes of Age   11
3 The Consultation   17
4 About Hospitals   33
5 The Facelift   39
6 Improving the Chin and the Jaw   71
7 Eyelid Surgery   89
8 Rhinoplasty: Reshaping the Nose   115
9 Chemabrasion and Dermabrasion   153
10 The Forehead and Brow Lift   183
11 Silicone and Collagen Treatments   195
12 Improving the Ear through Surgery   211
13 Hair Transplants   227
14 Uncommon Procedures and Developing Techniques   243
15 More Than Just a Pretty Face   251
Appendix: Chart   254
Index   257

Acknowledgments

The authors are most grateful to Richard M. Clurman for arranging their collaboration and for his wisdom and valuable advice in the preparation of this manuscript; to Genevieve Young for her enthusiasm and encouragement when the idea for the book was conceived; to Fredrica Friedman for her painstaking guidance through every step of the editorial process, and for the good taste and high literary standards she brought to bear on the manuscript; to Karola Noetel for her hard work, sunny disposition, and flair for handling the many details involved in keeping the work on track and on schedule; and to Dr. Hans Neumann for his infinite patience, objectivity, and good humor as, from the wings, he lent his support to the work in progress.

MORE THAN JUST A PRETTY FACE

"I never remember that anything beautiful, whether a man, a beast, a bird, or a plant, was ever shown, though it were to a hundred people, that they did not all immediately agree that it was beautiful."

— EDMUND BURKE, *A Philosophical Inquiry into Our Ideas of the Sublime and Beautiful*

"What is your fortune, my pretty maid?"
"My face is my fortune, sir," she said.
— NURSERY RHYME

Improving One's Looks: A Universal Desire | 1

BECAUSE YOU HAVE OPENED this book and are now reading these words, chances are that you have more than a passing interest in cosmetic surgery. Indeed, you may even have contemplated the possibility that such surgery might have something to offer you; that some small or larger feature which you consider unattractive, or perhaps some defect, could be corrected by a surgical procedure.

If you've had such thoughts, there's no reason for you to feel guilty or embarrassed because of them. I truly believe that most of us have, at one time or another, gazed into the mirror and contemplated the possibility of changing something about the way we look, or some feature of our faces or bodies. None of us is perfect; each of us can find some fault in our appearance even though it might be of a minor nature and our concern with it might perhaps be difficult for our friends or family to understand.

Each year, hundreds of thousands of people — men, women, and children — opt for some surgical procedure to improve their looks and, at the same time, raise their sense of self-esteem and confidence. Although cosmetic surgeries are not always reported to the American Society of Plastic and Reconstructive Surgeons (ASPRS) or to any other medical or government group, enough research has been done for us to have some reliable estimates on the number of people who undergo such operations. One indicator is the number of freestanding surgical centers — facilities that are not part of a hospital or doctor's office — in this country where three-quarters of all such procedures are performed.

By 1990, the number of freestanding surgical centers is expected to be close to 1,500, up from a mere 300 in 1984. It is anticipated that the amount of income for these centers will jump from about $226 million to $3.5 billion and that a considerable percentage of that figure will be paid out for cosmetic surgeries.

In 1984, the last year for which figures have, as yet, been compiled, the number of eyelid surgeries performed to correct bags and pouches under the eyes and on the upper eyelids had risen 31 percent in three years. There were recorded eyelid operations done on some 75,000 people, but so many more such procedures were probably performed which were not reported to the ASPRS that the true figure is probably over 100,000. We know that the frequency with which this operation is done has been growing rapidly and that, since the statistics were compiled in 1984, there has probably been another 30 percent increase.

People have flocked to surgeons for other facial cosmetic procedures as well. There are now between 75,000 and 100,000 nasal plastic surgeries being performed annually for cosmetic reasons. The number of chemical peels of the face to eliminate wrinkles has grown a big 67 percent between 1981 and 1984; and, annually, close to 30,000 people are undergoing chin augmentation. Cosmetic surgery has become the subject of numerous television specials and the popular magazines, not only those with female readerships, but also those that cater to male audiences, are finding that this subject is of wide popular interest.

No one foresaw this extraordinary growth in the relatively new specialty of cosmetic surgery, least of all those surgeons who pioneered the development of this burgeoning field during two World Wars. There is no other instance of such rapid development of a surgical specialty that can be used as a parallel.

Small wonder, since personal appearance, with emphasis on looks and youthfulness, has become so important to most of us. We live in an era when the maintenance of good health, physical and emotional, is a prime consideration for most informed and educated people in all advanced societies. We have learned that there are things we can do to stay well, to live longer, and to look better. Exercise, diet, cutting down or cutting out smoking, moderation in consuming alcoholic beverages, curtailing the exposure of our skin to direct sunlight, have become recognized factors in keeping our bodies healthy and attractive. Who, among all the people you know, would not choose to look younger, prettier, more handsome — given a choice?

While diet, exercise, and these other factors can go a long way towards improving one's health and appearance, they cannot alter certain facial features, such as the size and shape of the nose, a receded chin, or droopy eyelids. That's where cosmetic surgery comes in. Lending a hand to nature, modern surgery can go a long way towards enhancing one's looks — be it the nose, the chin, the eyes, the skin, or the ears that need help.

Cosmetic surgery, where indicated and when properly performed, does a great deal more than deliver just a pretty (or handsome) face. Thousands of people who have had successful facial surgery to improve their looks have reported that the changes resulting from such operations have made them happier than they had ever thought possible. Shy people have become outgoing, more social. Self-conscious people have grown self-confident, able to achieve in their careers and personal lives many goals they had previously found unattainable. Older people have regained their youthfulness, embarked on life-styles they once thought were behind them. A prettier, more handsome face has made some people walk taller, relate better, achieve more. The expression I hear most from patients after successful cosmetic surgery is *self-esteem*. "My self-esteem," they say, "is so vastly increased that I feel as though I'm beginning life all over again — this time with a face that's more to my liking."

The explosive growth of cosmetic surgery in recent years is also the result of widespread public acceptance of such surgery as a means of improving the quality of life; and, probably of equal importance, the acceptance by the medical fraternity at large that elective, cosmetic surgery is a legitimate method of providing "healing," even though it is, technically speaking, nonessential to the life or physical health of the individual electing to have it done. Modern surgery and anesthesia have become so safe for the elective and nonessential operation that the risks are negligible. The medical profession has accepted this fact and has come to embrace the new belief that the role of modern medicine should not be limited to the treatment of organic disease but should alleviate human suffering in all forms.

Yet another reason for the growth of this medical specialty is the rapid rate at which improvements in skill and technology have taken place in a relatively short period of time. On the other hand, plastic surgery has also become more complex, so that many surgeons subspecialize in microsurgery, aesthetic surgery, or reconstruction of defects resulting from burns, trauma, birth deformities, or other deviations from what we consider "normal."

All of these factors have contributed to making cosmetic surgery a widely acceptable route to improved looks and greater contentment, if not actual happiness.

I said up front that most of us have, at some point, considered the possibility of changing one thing or another about the way we look and that this is nothing to feel uncomfortable about. If you're contemplating an operation to improve your appearance, you will find many practical points of information in this book. Above all, you will learn the *truth* about cosmetic surgery — as best I can record it for you and as far as I am able to translate into nonscientific terms all of the information that this medical specialty has at its command.

Incidentally, in this book I will be using interchangeably the phrases *plastic surgery*, *cosmetic surgery*, and *aesthetic surgery*. The term *plastic surgery* is the oldest term and is commonly understood. However, it has nothing to do with plastic materials being used in this type of operation. The word *plastic* derives from the Greek word *plastikos,* meaning molded or shaped. I rather like the phrase *cosmetic surgery* because the word *cosmetic* relates to beauty as well as the correction of defects.

The greatest number of cosmetic surgery operations performed in this country and other advanced societies are for the correction of what might be considered purely aesthetic irregularities that are due either to our genes and heritage or to the aging process. And within *this* group, most involve facial surgery, surgery of the head: face, neck, ears, eyes, scalp. This book deals only with surgery on this part of the body and is basically for men and women of all ages who contemplate such surgery, or are close to a friend or relative for whom such surgery might be indicated.

I have tried to eliminate much of the mythology associated with cosmetic surgery, mythology that abounds in magazine articles and TV programs devoted to the subject. This book is based on my personal, hands-on experience of many years as a plastic surgeon. More than that, I believe that the viewpoints expressed here are shared by most, if not all, well-trained and Board Certified surgeons in this specialty who are trying to create the best possible improvement in each patient's appearance and, in so doing, bring them more than just a pretty face: help them find satisfaction with their looks and, with it, a feeling that life itself can, indeed, be beautiful.

I believe that, if truth were to be told, almost everyone in this day and age contemplates an aesthetic operation at various periods in life to improve his or her looks. Haven't you, yourself, looked in the mirror at some time during the past year and considered the possibility? Most people would have to answer that question with a "yes." The most beautiful people in the world, as well as those far less attractive, can find some physical feature in themselves that they don't like. Such imperfections, no matter how trivial, become increasingly difficult to accept with equanimity as one grows older. Aging is distressing to most people and it is quite normal to want to correct even small defects. Often, the people who tell you they "want to grow old gracefully" are concealing their true feelings about how they look. Some people just don't like to appear vain. Others feel that younger people, often their children, won't understand an aging person's desire to remain attractive. Those in the full bloom of youth find it difficult to think that *they* will ever be old — and even more difficult to believe they will ever *look* it.

Aging is difficult for everyone — anyone who tells you otherwise is masking a fear, or mouthing the clichés about contented old age in order to appear well adjusted. If aging is difficult for the average person in our society to accept, it is even more painful for those who have a huge nose, a receded chin, or some other obvious physical problem that has been a source of personal unhappiness over the years. While cosmetic surgery cannot stop the clock, it can put it on hold for a while; even set it back a few years. Surgery can blur the ravages of time, just as it can correct a physical deformity.

In the pages of a single book, it isn't possible for me to describe all the extraordinary and even miraculous accomplishments of which modern cosmetic surgery is capable. What this book will do is familiarize you with the basic procedures in facial surgery, give you more information than you might be able to get in a consultation with a busy practitioner, and answer the questions that you might feel reluctant to ask of a doctor you're meeting for the first time, and — perhaps as important as all the rest — debunk the many myths about cosmetic surgery that have sprung up over the years.

Of course, it would not be possible for me or any other surgeon to provide you with a total book of knowledge about any given procedure. If I could do that, we would then have to confer on every reader an honorary degree in plastic surgery. But I am certain you will come away from this book with enough information about cosmetic surgery in general, and about the particular operation you might be contemplating, to decide intelligently whether or not you want to pursue, in private consultation with an accredited surgeon, the possibility of having one or more surgical procedures performed.

A few words of caution up front: plastic surgery is not sculpting in clay or carving in wood. Human flesh is unique and individualistic. As surgeons, all we can do is trim away excess or rearrange the anatomical features available to us. Your surgeon cannot follow the blueprint of a photograph and reconstruct your face in the likeness of another image. People differ as well in their ability to heal, in the texture and elasticity of their skin, in their facial bone structures, in whether scars will be faint or marked, and in many other factors. Obviously, the surgeon seeks success every bit as much as the patient does. No one is happier than the surgeon when someone, through surgery, achieves the cosmetic results that were longed for before the operation.

What a skilled surgeon can accomplish is to make you look fresher, tidier, younger, *better*. He or she can trim down your nose if it is too large, or even change its angles — though he can't make you a new nose to order. No one should expect a so-called perfect result. If, in your fantasy, you are hoping that somewhere, somehow, someone can completely transform you, chances are you will be disappointed. I would urge anyone contemplating cosmetic surgery to be *realistic* — something I will say over and over again in this book. You are *you* — you will never become anyone else. Fortunately, most patients *are* realistic in their expectations and the vast majority of people who do have cosmetic surgery are more than pleased with the results.

On the subject of people wanting to be "transformed," I will tell you a true story. During World War II, three Norwegian patriots, well-known members of the underground movement in their country, were captured by the Gestapo but soon after managed to escape and make their way to England. These men were very valuable to the underground in Norway, as well as to Allied Intelligence. Once in England, they were taken by Allied Intelligence to a famous British plastic surgeon, Sir Archibald McIndoe, to undergo facial surgery in order for them to be able to return to Norway and continue in the resistance movement unrecognized by the enemy.

McIndoe used every technique known to camouflage the natural facial characteristics of these men. Despite extensive surgery, all three were recognized and recaptured by the Germans shortly after they returned to their homeland. It is extremely difficult, almost impossible, to alter facial characteristics so that people who know one well are unable to spot certain recognizable features. The most difficult thing to change is the look in one's eyes.

Soon after I opened my office in New York I was approached by two men who wanted me to "change the face" of one of their friends. The casting director for *The Godfather* would have picked these two men as perfect stereotypes for roles as members of the Mafia. It didn't take too much deduction on my part to figure out that their "friend" was probably a fugitive from the law.

I asked how they came by the idea that such an operation could be performed successfully, and they told me that they had heard about a book on the life of Sir Archibald McIndoe, who they had been told was my former mentor, which said that he had done such operations on the faces of some Norwegian spies during the Big War. What they hadn't known was the ultimate fate of those patriots. I tried to convince them that facial transformation through surgery, sufficient to completely disguise one's identity, was just not possible. They thought I was lying to them. They said they knew it *was* possible. Despite their not-so-veiled threats about what could be done to convince me to operate on their friend, I refused to undertake such an operation. To my enormous relief, they gave up and left my office — possibly to seek out some other surgeon who would do their bidding.

Cosmetic surgery, in and of itself, will not transform you. It cannot make you look like Cheryl Tiegs or Tom Selleck. On the other hand, it *can* make you look so much better, so much more attractive, so much more *to your own liking*, that your whole personality can be transformed. Sometimes, the change in a person's looks is so spectacular that he or she truly blossoms. I have seen men change from shy, insecure, even withdrawn personalities to friendly, outgoing people; I have seen women transformed from self-effacing, socially uncomfortable, and often timid people into jolly, warm, and confident achievers. As you read on, you will learn what cosmetic surgery *can* do to improve your looks . . . and how it *can* give you *more than just a pretty face*. Then, if you get to the point where you feel that cosmetic surgery may well be for you, ask yourself, "Why not?"

"It is not that that which is beautiful pleases us, but that that which pleases us is called beautiful."

— JEWISH PROVERB

Cosmetic Surgery Comes of Age | 2

"BEAUTY," SAID MARGARET WOLFE HUNGERFORD, "is in the eye of the beholder." The evidence is clear that man's concept of beauty has changed through the ages and it is likely to continue to do so for the rest of man's tenure on earth. The art of body adornment with paints and scarification dates from ancient times, probably from when the primitive man first discovered the unusual effects that result from smearing the body with mud or painting it with pigments. He may have discovered this by looking at his image in the original looking glass — a pond of water.

Adornment of the self through the use of cosmetics, clothes, hairstyles, or jewelry is widely accepted today, but the ancient tribal customs of scarification and tattooing are generally unacceptable in modern culture. Scarification in our society is generally considered to be a form of self-mutilation, usually indicating psychopathology. Tattooing is still a widespread form of decoration, but it is seen as being in bad taste, socially, in most advanced societies.

Thus, primitive man incises, paints, and decorates himself as an acceptable social form of ego manifestation, whereas modern "civilized" man is permitted only lesser degrees of self-adornment. What is socially acceptable can clearly mean different things in different cultures, at different times. Greek mythology tells us about a band of fierce women, the Amazons, who amputated their right breasts lest they interfere with drawing the bow. Tight chest binding was in vogue in ancient Hellenistic circles; it was thought to improve élan and poise. It came into vogue again in Chaucer's day and again in the 1920s. The small, firm breast, as opposed to the voluptuous breast popularized by some movie stars, became fashionable again in the early 1970s, and it is not inconceivable that breast binding could some day become fashionable once again, if not in our culture, then in others. Tight corsets were in vogue in the late nineteenth century to produce the "wasp waist."

There is considerable evidence to suggest that in pre-Columbian culture, people with harelip, dwarfism, and spinal deformities (such as hunchback) were revered and even accorded special privileges. Various deforming incisions were made in virtually every part of the body to enhance a popular concept of beauty in Africa, Asia, and the South Pacific, where such practices persist to this day.

Creating perforations of the nose, ears, cheeks, and lips, through which various articles of adornment such as shells, wooden plugs and stakes, precious and semi-precious stones, and, more recently, metals of different types could be worn, is also an ancient and widespread custom. Even in higher cultures, such as those of India and China, nose and ear perforation for the wearing of jewelry was a highly acceptable form of self-adornment.

The use of makeup was probably one of the first forms of self-decoration. Cosmetics, particularly facial, were highly developed and socially acceptable among the upper classes in ancient Crete. It should, therefore, surprise no one that body painting has recently enjoyed a brief vogue.

Very small, deformed feet resulted from the centuries-old tradition in China of binding the feet of female children. Such feet seem grotesque to most of us, but they were considered highly erotic by the Chinese men. Although officially outlawed by modern Chinese governments, foot binding died hard and slowly, in part because bound feet made walking difficult and served to keep women virtually in bondage. Yet even today, women with small, deformed feet can still be seen in Taiwan and the People's Republic.

Vanity, it would seem, is shared by all members of the human race, despite differences imposed by genetics, religion, geography, or historical custom. And why not? As patient after patient has said to me, "If I can look better, why shouldn't I?"

Yet cosmetic surgery as a commonly accepted branch of medicine in Western societies is a relatively new development. Plastic surgery was shrouded in secrecy until well into the third decade of this century. Today, it is out in the open as an accepted, often recommended, branch of medicine and a form of self-improvement that is growing by leaps and bounds. I mean that literally — it has leaped ahead of other forms of elective surgery and bounded into the mainstream of medicine with a rapidity unmatched in the annals of surgical specialties.

Aesthetic facial surgery was already being performed at the turn of this century, mostly by European surgeons who practiced their art in utter secrecy behind locked doors. Other surgeons were not permitted in their operating rooms. Rarely did they publish or write about their work, for they preferred not to share their knowledge with other plastic surgeons and certainly not with the medical community at large. When some material did see publication, it was often misleading — sometimes deliberately so. Important details were left out and imaginary operations were fantasized, even illustrated, in articles and books. Some of these published procedures were not only ineffective but downright dangerous, were a surgeon to follow them. This almost paranoid secrecy stemmed largely from two concerns: a fear of professional ostracism and an unwillingness to share a lucrative source of income.

Those who were able to break into this field did so through surgical lore and an accumulation of details picked up here and there from a small nucleus of people willing to talk about their successes and failures. This secrecy continued well into the 1930s. Some degree of it went on for two decades after that. I knew some of the pioneer aesthetic surgeons in New York very well. Almost all of them had European backgrounds, and because of their European traditions it was quite natural for them to remain secretive about their work. Many of these surgeons, in the old country, had paid their teachers considerable sums of money for the privilege of observing their operating techniques. The master surgeon who is credited with having developed *rhinoplasty*, Dr. Jacques Joseph of Berlin, charged his students several thousand dollars to observe him in the operating room — a custom not formerly uncommon between master craftsmen and apprentices.

The surgeons whom I observed early in my career, in the fifties, had paid for their training in this manner, and so they didn't consider it out of order to forbid observers in their operating rooms. Their demeanor to colleagues was always courteous, but distant and formal. And if you were a surgeon from the New York area, it was additionally difficult to gain admittance to their operating rooms because New York was where plastic surgery was developing and it presented a particular threat to those already ensconced in the specialty. You had to obtain a recommendation from a close friend of the surgeon even for permission to watch an operation, and asking questions about a technical point in the surgery was distinctly frowned upon. Often, the surgeon would block the observer's clear view of the operative field with a deft twist of the shoulder or the torso, making it impossible to observe the fine details and nuances of technique. Virtually all of this secrecy has been replaced in recent years by open communication and a willingness to share information within the medical field, with medical writers, and among laypersons. Today, experienced surgeons readily share their knowledge with interns, residents, and doctors in practice.

The public, however, loves an aura of mystery. People like to believe rumors that a certain surgeon in Paris, Rio de Janeiro, New York, or Timbuktu knows a very secret method of performing a facelift with virtually no scars — and that no other surgeon is privy to this knowledge. Many of these ridiculous tales are prompted by irresponsible magazine or newspaper writers, pandering to the guillibility of readers; or, I'm sorry to say, by professional public relations consultants trying to gain fame or notoriety for a doctor-client. Such stories are, of course, rubbish. There are no secret techniques or procedures in surgery today. Cosmetic surgery has come out of the closet and into the drawing room. Naturally, there are variations in performance, degrees of competence, and some physicians are more adept at certain procedures than are others. But secrets? There are none.

Everything is in the medical literature and no sooner does an improvement in technique evolve than someone has written a paper about it. I see nothing wrong in a patient wishing to travel to some city far from home in order to have an operation performed by the surgeon of his or her choice. But traveling to Brazil or Switzerland or Tahiti or anywhere else to search out a surgeon with a secret technique is nonsense.

The so-called jet-setters or beautiful people are usually personable, interesting, frequently talented, charming, and tasteful. They are often highly knowledgeable about what is happening in the world and especially about their own professions — which include the theater and television, movies, journalism, publishing, advertising, corporate affairs, government and politics, and fashion. Traveling is second nature to this group, and they will readily cross continents to seek out new medical treatments, whether it be cellular membrane injections in Switzerland or a visit to a highly touted plastic surgeon in Pago Pago.

Despite their knowledge and sophistication about most matters, the "beautiful people" often embrace the newest fad and follow their social leaders in matters relating to medicine and rejuvenation. The point I want to make is that simply because you read about such celebrities making a pilgrimage to some other country (often exotic) to get "cellular regeneration" shots, "youth injections," or even plastic surgery that employs "new" or "secret" techniques, does not mean that what you've read is necessarily correct, or that you should board the first available plane and follow along. As I have said before, there are no secret techniques in plastic surgery. Very likely, the latest advances are being practiced close to home, if not in your own hometown. All you need to do is locate a qualified surgeon.

The communications media, especially television, is a potent force in providing information to the general public. Now that so many people are living well beyond middle age, anything pertaining to medicine and nutrition is considered newsworthy. But because things pass so quickly on the TV screen, it's often impossible to go into great detail on any given subject. Frequently, all aspects of a subject are not fully explored. Thus, a brief comment on a news program, or a very short segment within a program, may fail to explain fully to the audience that some newly heralded procaine injection from Bulgaria, or some cellular injection therapy from the Bahamas, is unsupported by a single shred of scientific evidence about their efficacy.

Often, one will hear people comment that they believe a conspiracy exists between the medical profession and the Food and Drug Administration to prevent the American public from enjoying a new treatment or palliative because doctors are conservative, even reactionary, and they don't want to encourage the use of anything that will alter the status quo in terms of current treatment methods. This, of course, is such nonsense as to defy reason.

On the positive side, I can assure you that the vast majority of accredited plastic surgeons are competent, skilled professionals who are devoting the greater part of their lives to helping people solve those anatomical problems which are making them unhappy. They are dedicated to their careers and to their patients, and usually up to date on the latest techniques and surgical procedures that can contribute to the physical and psychological well-being of people who are unhappy with their looks.

At last count, there were 3,300 Board Certified plastic surgeons in this country. In addition, there are many physicians in other specialties — eye doctors, dermatologists, general surgeons, and ear, nose, and throat specialists — who also do cosmetic surgery. So, while I would advise you, if you are considering cosmetic surgery, to beware of so-called secret procedures, and of the rumor mill, no matter how much you revere the public personalities who feed it, I would also like to assure you that there is no shortage of skilled, trained, and well-qualified surgeons who can help you in your quest for improved or more youthful looks and, in so doing, give you more than just a pretty (or handsome) face.

Each of us has but one life to live on this earth, and we are entitled to live it in good health and good spirits, if at all possible. Since cosmetic surgery has come of age in this and most other developed societies, people who want their inner spirit of youthfulness to be matched by their outer appearance, or those who merely want to correct or improve some facial flaw in order to be more at peace with their looks, should feel comfortable in their desire to see a qualified surgeon and learn whether cosmetic surgery might help them achieve their goals.

"It is the common wonder of all men, how among so many millions of faces, there should be none alike."

— SIR THOMAS BROWNE, *Religio Medici*

The Consultation | 3

A CONSULTATION WITH A cosmetic surgeon is a unique experience. Though you've consulted with doctors before, with the exception of your annual physical examination, your visits concerned some medical problem for which you sought a diagnosis and treatment that would make you feel better. Now you're in a strange doctor's office as a healthy person who just wants to *look* better.

You may feel ill at ease, perhaps a bit defensive ("I'm not the only one who says I should get my nose fixed . . . my mother thinks . . ."); maybe a little apologetic ("I hate to sound so vain . . ."); and perhaps somewhat anxious ("I've been toying with this idea for years, so I don't know why I'm so nervous . . ."). Virtually all patients feel one or more of these emotions at the time of their first visit to a cosmetic surgeon.

One important purpose of a consultation is, however, to allay your fears and anxieties by helping you learn as much as possible about the surgery you have been contemplating. You should look on the consultation as a fact-finding mission. You have scheduled this meeting to learn all you can about cosmetic surgery, about the operation you may eventually undergo, and whether, realistically, you can hope to achieve the surgical results you want. True, as a potential patient for plastic surgery you probably want more than just a surgical procedure. While you do want surgical help with your facial problem, a rapid and uncomplicated recovery after surgery, and results as good as or better than you had hoped for, you probably also want a doctor who can understand your reasons for desiring the surgery and who offers you reassurance that the operation you are considering is a wise move. So, since you are going to entrust your health, your sense of well-being, and your *looks* to this doctor whom you barely know, you have a right to expect more than *facts* in your consultation.

I think it's very important for a patient to believe she or he has the "right" doctor because positive feelings are an important building block in creating a successful surgery. As the cofounder of the African Medical & Research Foundation, I spend a month every year in East Africa operating on adults and children with physical deformities that require plastic surgery, and I have come to know the people there very well. I have seen Africans recover from devastating illness because of faith in their witch doctors or because of the inner strength they are able to muster when trying to overcome pain and suffering. In less developed societies, the threshold of pain is much higher than in our culture because disease, death, hunger, and other problems are so much a part of the fabric of everyday life. Since true physical suffering, such as that experienced in some of the African tribes I know, is so rare in our advanced society, we have tuned down our natural apparatus for coping with it.

But we who are in medicine know that an optimistic patient who believes she or he is in good hands, with the "right," caring doctor, is an excellent candidate for quick recovery and satisfaction with the surgical results. So, another function of the consultation is to determine whether you feel that you and the surgeon have the right chemistry, the right rapport, for you to move towards a surgical procedure.

You should recognize, however, that while the initial impressions you gain in a first consultation are important, they sometimes alter after a second or perhaps third meeting. So don't be too quick to judge the doctor or the relationship between the two of you. If his answers to your questions are short, to the point, maybe even blunt, it could be because he knows his subject matter so well he takes it for granted you know more about aesthetic surgery than you actually do. It would be a mistake to jump to the conclusion that concise answers mean the doctor is unfeeling, too hurried, or that he dislikes you. None of this may be the case. A consultation with a plastic surgeon is one instance where first impressions can be completely wrong and change 180 degrees in a second meeting.

Negative feelings sometimes arise because so many physicians are brilliant in their specialties but poor as communicators. Beyond their medical specialties, they also specialize in repeating to you in Greek what you just told them in English.

Examples: PATIENT: "I'm depressed by these tiny crow's-feet around my eyes."
DOCTOR: "You have developed rhytides." [Greek for wrinkles or crow's-feet.]

PATIENT: "Doctor, my hair is falling out."
DOCTOR: "You are suffering from alopecia." [Greek for falling hair.]

If you do feel uncomfortable with the surgeon you've consulted, ask for a follow-up consultation with him or a member of his staff. You may find that your initial discomfort was not so much due to poor chemistry as to the general unease that sometimes occurs when discussing intimate feelings about appearance with a total stranger, albeit a physician. Very often, the relationship thaws with the greater familiarity of a second consultation.

If, however, after a second consultation, you still feel uneasy about the relationship and question whether you want this doctor to operate on you, by all means seek an opinion from another qualified surgeon. But I would caution you against too many consultations and opinions — you could end up very confused. If the doctor or doctors you see are well qualified, then you certainly do not need more than two opinions, unless you happen to have an extraordinarily unique problem where a superspecialist might be called for.

I've said that the consultation is a fact-finding expedition for you. But every consultation is different. It is a highly individualized procedure. Were a surgeon to tape a dozen interviews with patients considering nose surgery, no two would be alike. It is quite a different consultation from that which a cardiac or cancer surgeon might have with a patient, in which surgical treatment for an illness is discussed. What you're contemplating is a purely elective procedure and the information you come away with will help you decide whether you want to go ahead with it.

What You Should Learn in a Consultation

Speaking broadly, what you should learn in a first or second consultation is whether the condition for which you sought a surgeon's opinion is correctible through cosmetic surgery, whether you are a suitable candidate for the contemplated operation, whether you are seeking help with your problem at the right time in your life, how realistic your goals are apropos of the surgery, and what you can anticipate in terms of time, pain, inconvenience, and money. And, of course, as I have pointed out, how you feel about the particular doctor you've consulted. You will also want to learn in the consultation if there is any down side to the surgery in terms of possible complications and, if so, how serious and how common such complications are likely to be.

Are Your Expectations Realistic?

In the first chapter of this book I urged anyone contemplating cosmetic surgery to be realistic in terms of his or her expectations about what such surgery might accomplish. I consider this a critical factor in whether or not someone will be happy with the results of a cosmetic operation, and it's something you should give a good deal of thought to before you have your consultation. It is also something that you should explore with the surgeon in your very first meeting.

Cosmetic surgery is a combination of art and science. From a scientific point of view, the surgeon brings to the operating room his training, knowledge, and experience with the procedure you will undergo. You can assume that a qualified, Board Certified physician is up to the minute on the state of the art for such surgery.

But there is also a great deal of artistry brought to this specialty by the surgeon. The degree to which a doctor can mold and sculpt tissue and bone into pleasing and agreeable forms is what distinguishes a good surgeon from a great one. It is upon such talents that surgeons' reputations are often built.

But human tissue differs person to person. The results achieved in one patient cannot always be duplicated in another. Even the finest surgeon, respected by his peers, with many hundreds of successful cases to his credit, is not capable of turning you into someone else, or re-creating your face in such ways as will make you into the person you would like to be. He can, perhaps, to some degree, tighten your jawline, remove bags and pouches from your eyes, make your ears protrude less, provide you with a suitably attractive nose to replace the one you don't like, remove or eliminate certain wrinkles — all this is possible.

However, what you must do in a consultation is explore with your surgeon what you hope to accomplish through a cosmetic procedure — and then ask him if your goal is a realistic one. Perhaps he will say "yes." But be prepared that he may, on the other hand, tell you that your expectations will not be wholly fulfilled. In that case, ask him what you *can* expect the surgery to do for you. Should you determine from his answer that such a result would not make you happy, you might be better off postponing surgery until such time as you can come to terms with a more realistic goal. Possibly cosmetic surgery is not for you, although it has been my experience that normally healthy people, when they learn what an operation can be expected to do for them, will accept a specialist's evaluation.

PREPARING FOR THE CONSULTATION

Many patients arrive at a consultation unclear about what they hope to gain by the surgery, and their questions are so open-ended as to make it difficult and time-consuming for the surgeon to get down to what the patient sees as the problem.

A good technique to help clarify in your own mind what you hope to achieve through surgery is to write down what bothers you, being as specific as possible. The best way to do this is to look in the mirror and see what truly troubles you, then put it down on paper. For example, if you want to modify a large nose, it would be helpful to the surgeon to know whether it's your profile or the front view of your face that troubles you most; or whether it's the bridge or the tip that you see as unattractive.

Often it's difficult to define the anatomical correction that you are seeking. While some deformities are instantly obvious to both the patient and doctor, there are certain signs of aging, subtle but indefinable changes in the face, that are difficult to explain. In preparing yourself for the consultation with written notes, you will have time at home, alone, to analyze your feelings about your looks and crystallize your thinking. This, at minimum, gives you a starting point for your consultation. When the surgeon opens with a question such as "Well, what can I do for you?" or "What troubles you?" you'll know where to start.

It helps to be specific, if you can. The patient who says, "What can you do for me, doctor, I don't like my looks" is not a very good candidate for surgery. She doesn't know what her specific objectives are in terms of a surgical procedure. Does she want to look younger? Fresher? Less haggard? Or does she want to look like someone else — perhaps her sister or a celebrity whose looks she admires?

The patient who says, "I'm bothered by my sagging neck" or "These bags under my eyes began to appear about a year ago. I'd like to eliminate them, if possible" is a much better candidate for surgery.

What Doesn't Help in the Consultation

Frequently, patients arrive with photographs of themselves at a younger age (often it's a wedding picture) or of movie stars or other celebrities, in the mistaken belief that a surgeon can re-create their faces in the image of an expectantly tendered photo. The patient who brings many photographs, particularly if they are of other people, worries the physician because he knows that it's exceedingly rare for a surgical procedure to create a new face, or even a new nose, according to design specifications.

On the other hand, photographs can sometimes be helpful if they show explicitly what the patient does *not* like. In such instances, a picture can be worth a thousand words.

Another form of preparation for your first visit with the surgeon which doesn't help much, if at all, is to read a lot of articles on aesthetic surgery. Unless you know that an article was written by an established and reputable cosmetic surgeon or science writer, you run the risk of picking up a few facts and a good deal of fiction. This is not to say that some of the more respected magazines haven't, at times, run some excellent articles on the subject. They have. But I have also seen articles that fall into the category of "sensational journalism" which have been full of misinformation. If you think enough of a surgeon to want to consult with him, let him answer your questions. He will, very likely, also provide you with literature that will fill in the informational gaps.

If you have read some articles, and if they make you want to ask questions during your consultation, write down the questions rather than arriving at the doctor's office with the article itself, or with an open-ended scenario on what you plan to discuss.

Physical and Psychological Assessment

After the doctor has discussed with you the problem that brought you to his office and offered some feedback on whether he thinks your goals are realistic, the consultation will probably move on to a physical evaluation to determine whether cosmetic surgery can completely or partially correct your problem. The doctor will examine your face from the front and side view; he may take some measurements of one or more parts of your face; if your eyes are the organs to be operated on, he may ask his nurse or assistant to give you an eye test; and he will also take your medical history. Such history is often taken by means of a questionnaire which you might be asked to fill out in the waiting room, or taken down by a nurse or secretary when you arrive at the office. When the doctor examines you, he will then ask you additional questions.

You will be asked what medication you are on, if any; whether you smoke; how much alcohol you consume; about any bleeding problems you may ever have experienced; what allergies you have, and so on. You will very likely be asked the same questions again when you enter the hospital or clinic for surgery — not by your surgeon but by a nurse or resident physician. You may wonder why the surgeon didn't send a copy of your medical history to the hospital and eliminate the need for a second, similar history-taking. The principal reason is that the hospital wants to have its own record, taken by one of its staff members, on its own form — otherwise they'd be dealing with forms and formats from a large number of doctors, each of whom has his own style (sometimes a personal form of shorthand) for obtaining patient information.

During the consultation, the surgeon will also make a psychological assessment of your attitude towards your problem. While cosmetic surgeons are not trained specifically in the techniques of psychiatric evaluation, they come to know, after hundreds of patient interviews, when someone's objectives in seeking surgery have not been soundly and seriously thought through. In such cases, the physician will often provide a patient with literature to read at home and will suggest a second consultation, either with himself or another member of the staff.

The psychological assessment is quite important, since the doctor will want to recommend for or against aesthetic surgery and he needs to know what's in your mind regarding this subject, as well as what he can see on your face. He will have to make his decision in a relatively short period of time (a surgeon and his patient are not in a long-term psychiatric relationship), so most experienced surgeons develop an extrasensory perception that alerts them to the need for an additional consultation, a need to wait some months to see if the desire for surgery persists, or a flat (but considerate) refusal to perform the operation.

Formulating Your Questions

You have a right to expect that all your pertinent questions will be answered in the consultation, either by the physician, his staff, or through printed material he will give you. It helps if you try to make your questions direct, brief and specific.

Let me suggest the type of questions that are appropriate in a consultation. No two patients bring precisely the same problem, combined with the same level of knowledge and sophistication, to the consulting room. Therefore, some of the following questions may not necessarily be ones that you will want to ask — you may already know the answers to them. In some instances, the literature the nurse gives you to read while you're waiting to see the doctor will already have answered the questions. But it will help clarify your own thinking if you write down your questions in advance of the consultation; or, at minimum, come to the fact-finding session with a few notes that will remind you of the questions you want to ask.

Typical Questions

Here are the questions I'm asked most frequently during consultations.

Am I a suitable candidate for the surgery I'm interested in? Is my problem one that can be improved or corrected by such a surgical procedure?

On a scale of one to ten, can I expect a result that would be nine or ten? Or is it more likely to be three or four?

Is this the proper time in my life to have this surgery or should I wait?

[When a facelift is contemplated] Would I be better off having it done in a few years?

Is the operation painful?

Is there much pain or discomfort *after* the operation? How long?

What type of anesthesia do you recommend for this operation?

What are the advantages and disadvantages of the general anesthesia versus the local anesthesia?

Is there a difference in cost between the two types?

Will my surgery be done in a hospital or in an office or an ambulatory center?

Am I safer in one or the other facility?

What is the difference in cost between the hospital and the ambulatory center?

If I have it done on an ambulatory basis, who will take care of me immediately after the surgery?

Will I need certain care after the surgery which is easier to get in the hospital than if I go right home from an ambulatory facility?

Does my insurance cover any part of the operation: your fee, the anesthesia, the hospital or ambulatory charges?

How long will I have to stay out of work and out of social functions? Full time out of work? Part time out of work?

After how many days am I likely to feel comfortable in a social setting?

How many months does the entire healing process take?

What can I expect during this healing period?

Will there be marks or scars from the surgery?

[If so,] Where will they be located?

Will they be very noticeable? Will they interrupt or interfere with my life in any way?

Are such marks or scars permanent? Do they get better as time goes on?

What complications can occur in the surgery I'm thinking of?

Are these complications common or rare? Are they serious?

What are the down-side risks in such surgery?

If the results of my operation are not entirely to my satisfaction, can it be repeated or done over?

If the procedure is repeated, what chances for success are there the second time around?

What are the expenses involved in a corrective procedure?

Do I pay a second fee to you? For the anesthesia? For the hospital or ambulatory facility?

Are any of these costs covered by insurance?

Are the costs of either the first or second procedure tax-deductible?

Does your fee include postoperative care? Does it include treatment for complications, should they arise?

Based on your experience with other patients, can you tell me what to expect in terms of reactions from friends and colleagues?

Should I tell my immediate family I'm going to have this surgery? What about my co-workers?

Can you show me any photos of patients before and after their surgery, so I can get an idea of what I might expect?

How soon after this surgery can I bathe? Wash my hair? Apply makeup? Do physical exercise?

How soon after the surgery can I have sex?

How Long a Consultation Lasts

I've just given you a long list of questions that are appropriate for a patient to ask a surgeon or a member of his staff. Were every patient to ask a doctor all of those questions and be given complete answers, that doctor would be able to interview very few patients and still have time to do any surgery. However, as I pointed out, not all of those questions are for all patients; and many of them will be answered by a member of the doctor's staff, or in the literature he gives you to read.

Speaking very generally, most consultations last between fifteen minutes and three-quarters of an hour. Every doctor has his own style of consulting, so no one can set a hard and fast timetable to this fact-finding session. Few surgeons personally answer all the routine questions (such as those about fees, insurance, when to resume work or exercise, or the use of makeup). Most surgeons concentrate on answering those questions directly related to the surgical process itself, the likelihood of achieving the desired results, and the patient's suitability for the operation. Another staff member usually answers the other questions.

All in all, combining the time spent in giving a medical history, being examined by the surgeon, and the follow-up discussion with a member of the staff, you will probably spend an hour or more in the doctor's office when you go for your initial consultation. How long the session lasts is less important than what you learn from it.

Expressing Your Doubts

I would urge you to speak freely to your doctor. If you have any doubts about whether surgery is for you, don't hesitate to express them during the consultation. With rare exceptions, patients always have some doubts or mixed feelings on the subject of an elective operation. If your doubts are very strong and outbalance your motivation for wanting the surgery, the doctor may recommend that you wait a while until your feelings have sorted themselves out. By the time you have a second consultation, probably some months in the future, you are likely to have a more clearly defined picture of what you hope to achieve through cosmetic surgery and why you've had doubts about it.

Don't try to read the doctor's mind. A patient in such doubting circumstances might think, "Oh-oh! I've talked him out of wanting to redo my nose — after waiting all these weeks to see him." Not at all. The doctor, sensing the strength of your doubts, may feel it's in your own best interests to let the idea of surgery perk a little longer. When you are certain this is the route you want to take, he'll probably have no qualms about booking you for an operation if other pertinent factors also point in that direction.

On Listening to the Answers

I'm sure you've had the experience of having someone ask you a question and then not pay much attention when you answer it. Occasionally we all do that. But it is particularly true during medical consultations. A patient will ask a question and then, out of nervousness or in the interest of saving the doctor's time, will be so busy formulating the next question that the answer to the first one is not fully absorbed. Furthermore, when the information being given has to do with an unpleasant subject, such as the possibility of surgical complications, people often practice "selective listening" — they hear only what they want to hear.

I would, therefore, urge you to try and relax during the consultation and absorb as much of the information as you can.

Informed Consent

Unfortunately, many people believe that surgery — not only for aesthetic purposes, but all surgery — is an exact science and that it should be perfect, without risk, and that mishaps should never occur. This attitude is fostered by attorneys specializing in malpractice cases and has led to laws in the United States (but in very few other countries) where patients must give their doctor a signed paper stating that they have been informed about all possible risks involved in their specific surgery, and that they are consenting to such surgery fully aware of the risks they are undertaking.

Some surgeons have such long, detailed consent forms they read like legal documents full of fine print, and patients, if they want the operation, are compelled to sign them before surgery. Other surgeons — and I am one of them — give their patients a paper designed to provide them with as much practical information as is possible without scaring them half to death about the multitude of complications (most of them highly unlikely) that could befall them. While good sense dictates that enough information should be given to all patients so they know what to expect, it's simply not possible to give everyone a complete course in medicine and surgery.

If you are asked to sign such an informed-consent paper before surgery, know that it's part of today's medical system, required by certain laws and insurance companies, and that it doesn't mean you're in terrible danger.

Checking the Doctor's Credentials

If you want to research a doctor's credentials before making an appointment to see him, go to the library and look in a book called the *Marquis Who's Who Directory of Medical Specialists*. In the section on plastic surgeons, you'll probably find the name of the doctor you're considering — if, of course, he is qualified. If he or she is a medical doctor (M.D.) and is a Diplomate in Plastic Surgery (D.P.S.), it means that the physician has been "certified" by the American Board of Plastic Surgery ("Board Certified"). This tells you that the doctor was specially trained in general surgery for three to five years and spent a minimum of two more years training in an approved plastic surgery program in a hospital or a teaching center. To obtain certification, a plastic surgeon, after all the years of training, must also pass rigorous oral and written examinations in plastic surgery. So, if he or she has passed the "Boards" and is "Certified," you know that, at least, they've had the right training.

There are other surgeons, besides plastic surgeons, who are also qualified to do cosmetic surgery. Eye specialists (ophthalmologists) do eyelid surgery; ear, nose, and throat specialists (otolaryngologists, known as ENT specialists) do nose and sometimes facial surgery; and specially trained dermatologists do dermabrasion and chemabrasion, as well as hair transplants. The same *Directory of Medical Specialists* will give you the credentials of physicians in these other specialties.

The American Society of Plastic and Reconstructive Surgeons, Inc., was formed some years ago to promote optimal care for plastic surgery patients through education, research, and high professional standards. The society is located at 233 North Michigan Avenue, Suite 1900, Chicago, IL 60601, and their toll-free number is 800-635-0635 (in Illinois, 312-856-1834). Should you seek information you can't find in the library, a call to the society might help you in your research.

Discussing Fees and Other Costs

Most physicians assign someone on their staff — a secretary, a nurse, an administrator, or assistant — the responsibility of discussing with you the matter of the doctor's fee, hospital charges, the anesthesiologist's fee, the cost of preoperative and postoperative medical photos, and other costs that you might incur, such as the cost of an EKG or chest X ray that your particular hospital might require upon admission.

Among the questions I listed before that are appropriate for a patient to ask during a consultation were some involving fees and charges. If neither the doctor nor his nurse mentions fees and costs, be certain that you bring it up. This is important information for you to carry away from the consultation. Since cosmetic surgery is an elective procedure, there is usually no urgency in making a date for the operation. So, if you want to think about the fees and other costs before committing yourself to a surgical appointment, feel free to say, "I'd like to think about that and I'll call you when I've made up my mind."

Making the Decision

Finally, though the surgeon you've selected may feel that you are a suitable candidate for a specific surgical procedure and assure you that the results will very likely be what you are hoping for, the ultimate decision on whether to go ahead with the operation is up to you. Only you know how strongly motivated you are, how troubled you are by some facial flaw or sign of aging. And only you know whether you are willing and able to spare the time, spend the money, and possibly experience some pain or discomfort, in order to achieve a specific cosmetic improvement in your appearance.

If you are like the vast majority of people who have had cosmetic surgery, the chances are excellent that the results of your own aesthetic procedure will leave you feeling that you're beginning life anew, or that you've managed to trim away the evidence of your aging. You can then go forward in life with improved looks and the improved spirits that almost always accompany such a change for the better.

About Hospitals | 4

*E*VERYTHING YOU'VE EVER heard about hospitals is true — in some measure, in some places, in some ways, in some circumstances.

Going into a hospital is not a joyous experience. Hospitals are full of sick people, strange smells, long corridors, and noisy nights.

All of us have heard our share of horror stories about hospitals: nurses waking you from a deep sleep to give you a sleeping pill, aides skipping your room when they make their rounds with the breakfast trays, missing X rays, roommates with loud and inconsiderate visitors, and all the rest.

Many of these stories are exaggerated; for the sake of a good tale, raconteurs often embellish the truth. But many such things *do* happen. Running a hospital is not an exact science, and a lot depends upon the personnel a hospital can attract. However, if you decide to have cosmetic surgery and if you have it done as an in-hospital patient, remember that you're going into the hospital as a *well* person, on an elective basis, and your psychological and physical resources are much better than those of a patient who had no choice about being hospitalized, and who may be there for treatment of a serious or debilitating illness.

Nowadays, many hospitals "preregister" patients. They send

you a form to fill out with vital statistics and return to them so that, when you enter the hospital for surgery, you will have been computerized and, theoretically at least, you won't have to cool your heels while the admitting office prepares the paperwork on your case. Some hospitals send with the form to be filled out a piece of promotional literature that tells you what a great hospital you're about to enter. "You are about to become a patient in a very special hospital," it may inform you; or "We are known the world over for our excellent patient care and a friendly, helpful atmosphere"; or "Our entire staff is dedicated to making you comfortable and well." Maybe so; maybe not. That copy has probably been written by someone in the public relations department who's never been hospitalized, so take it with a grain of salt. If it all turns out to be true, count your blessings.

It's generally said that the big-city "teaching" hospitals have access to the newest equipment and procedures and that they attract the best interns and residents to their staff. The other side of the coin is that small-town hospitals are said to have dedicated, friendly, "local" help on the nonmedical staff and that such people are more inclined to be patient and relaxed with their charges. As with all generalities, these concepts about small-town vs. big-city hospitals have so many exceptions as to make them almost invalid. But you know your own city or town, so you probably know what to expect when you're hospitalized.

The best advice I can give you is in two parts. First, anticipate that your stay in the hospital will not be akin to a stay at your favorite luxury resort — at best it will be routine and uneventful; at worst it will provide you with enough anecdotal material to dine out on for months to come. Second, keep your sense of humor about your hospital stay. Being able to chuckle, if not actually laugh, about glitches in your hospital confinement will keep you on an even keel and enhance your recovery.

You can expect the very best care from everyone when you're actually in the operating and recovery rooms. Despite what the TV comedies may tell you, procedures in every accredited hospital are medically approved, scientifically correct, and carefully monitored by state and local boards. If you go into an accredited hospital or clinic and are operated on by an accredited surgeon, relax . . . you're in good hands.

And stay sunny. A patient who is of good cheer is already on the way to successful surgery and a speedy, uncomplicated recovery.

The Alternative — Outpatient Surgery

If you don't want your surgery done in a hospital, you belong to a big club — and a growing one. Operating in the hospital may not be your surgeon's choice, either. An increasing number of plastic surgery procedures are being performed on an outpatient, or "ambulatory," basis in surgical centers that are either freestanding or connected with a hospital. Many plastic surgeons have their own operating suites, completely independent of any hospital setting, while many hospitals are now busy building such "surgicenters" for one-day surgery.

The principal reason for this trend away from in-hospital surgery is to keep down medical costs. It's expensive to run a hospital, and when you, the patient, get your bill, all of the hospital's built-in costs and expenses have been averaged out — and you or your insurance carrier is picking up part of that tab. Since elective plastic surgery is not covered by many insurance policies or by Medicare, it's most often the patient who pays this bill, and the difference in cost between a night or two in the hospital and the use of an outpatient operating facility can be substantial.

There are other reasons why many patients and surgeons prefer outpatient surgery: it minimizes inconvenience to both of them; it cuts down on time lost; and there's usually a difference in atmosphere and environment between a hospital room and one in a surgicenter. Freestanding facilities are usually decorated to provide a restful, even attractive, environment in which a patient who is not really sick can find comfort and reassurance. Hospital rooms, by contrast, do tend to intimidate, even frighten, some patients.

Surgeons have embraced the concept of outpatient surgery because so many patients for elective operations are less apprehensive in a nonhospital setting, prefer the idea of going home to convalesce, and are happy to enjoy the savings realized by the one-day surgery procedure as contrasted to the cost of one or more nights in a hospital.

Because outpatient surgical units are relatively new, there are not, as yet, any uniform regulations that have been adopted nationwide. Some states do have regulations regarding these surgical centers, and some insurance companies have established standards that must be met before they will provide insurance coverage for them. There are also some independent organizations that are now certifying surgical clinics if they meet a given set of standards. One such group is the Association of Ambulatory Surgery Facilities, which provides a certification to a unit if it passes a stringent on-site investigation by the association's inspectors and is found to be worthy of accreditation. Such on-site examination of an outpatient facility assures, at least, that it has state-of-the-art equipment and safety precautions.

A proper ambulatory surgical facility should include these features: a reception area; a dressing room; an inner waiting room for the family of someone in surgery; an operating suite that consists of an operating room or rooms, as well as a dressing room (known as a "sterilizing area") in which the staff can change into sterile clothes. A properly equipped recovery room is also a requirement.

Of prime importance is the presence of all forms of equipment that insure safety for patients. This equipment is usually the same as is found in hospitals and, in some instances, may be even more elaborate. Included are such things as EKG monitors, pulse monitors, resuscitation equipment, anesthesia machinery, an oxygen source, and an emergency lighting source, such as a generator.

It is also necessary for an ambulatory unit to have access to a proper blood bank and an agreement with the local hospital to accept, without question, any patient who might experience an emergency requiring more intensive and prolonged care.

The personnel of an ambulatory surgical unit is also an important factor. There must be, of course, a qualified surgeon and perhaps a surgical assistant in attendance at all surgical procedures, as well as registered nurses in both the operating suite and the recovery room. Sometimes a nurse, a surgical technician, as well as an anesthetist, is also employed by some ambulatory clinics.

If you opt for surgery on an ambulatory basis, be sure that the facility recommended by your doctor is a proper surgical unit that meets your state's safety requirements, or that it has been certified by an organization such as the Association of Ambulatory Surgery Facilities. Don't be embarrassed to ask your surgeon, or his nurse or secretary, whether the recommended facility has been certified by any local or regional evaluating group. If the answer you get is a mere "Yes, it has been," feel free to ask for the name of the certifying organization. If there is any doubt in your mind, call your local county medical association and ask for an opinion on the certifying group. While there's no need to be aggressive or rude in your questioning, it's *your* face, *your* health, and *your* pocketbook that are at stake, so you have every right to find out all you can about the facility that's been recommended. Chances are that if the surgeon is a reputable one, his ambulatory surgical facility will be first-rate.

In any case, whether you go in-hospital or outpatient, you're going to be in and out before you know it. Almost all of your convalescence as a postoperative patient who's had cosmetic surgery is going to be at home, in an environment that is probably under your own control, at least to some degree.

And now, let me tell you everything you may want to know about the aesthetic surgeries performed most frequently.

"We ascribe beauty to that which is simple; which has no superfluous parts; which exactly answers its end; which stands related to all things; which is the mean of many extremes."

— R. W. EMERSON, *The Conduct of Life*

The Facelift | 5

A MONTH AFTER MY FACELIFT, *seated in a chair at my hairdresser's and wearing a salon smock that fully revealed my throat down to my collarbone, I glanced in the large mirror and saw with joy that the area of my body I was viewing was so youthful looking I could hardly believe it was me. The skin that had hung loosely beneath my jaw for several years was now attractively tight and, as I turned my face sidewards, I saw that the whole jawline looked clean and young. I felt a moment of sheer elation at the "new me" and I silently thanked my lucky stars that the preoperation fears and doubts I had experienced had not altered my decision to have a facelift.*

I recall the night before I was scheduled for surgery. It was after the visiting hours and I lay sleepless in my darkened room. There were dim lights in the corridor and low voices at the nurses' station down the hall. Suddenly, I was overcome with fear. I was alone in a city sixty miles from my hometown. The bed was too narrow and I missed my husband. Why, I thought, have I gotten myself into this? I'm a healthy, forty-nine-year-old woman . . . why did I go into a hospital to make myself sick? Why am I playing around with Mother Nature? Vanity brought me this far. Will vanity give me strength if something goes wrong? My fear escalated to terror. I had, until that moment, hidden from myself my fear of surgery, of the unknown, of being unconscious, of having anesthesia administered to me. I was afraid of pain, fearful I'd wake up in the recovery room, hurting.

Then I remembered the "before" photos that had been taken of me so that my surgeon could examine my face in detail, as the camera saw it. I thought about my creping neck, the "rooster" neck I hated so much, the fat under my chin, and the old-lady look I had come to dread when I looked in the mirror. I still thought of myself as a young woman, and I didn't want to see myself so aged, looking so worn-out.

I took three deep breaths and rang for the floor nurse. She came at once. "I would like a sleeping pill," I told her. "I'm apprehensive and I can't sleep." She brought me a red and yellow capsule and I soon dozed off. The next thing I knew it was dawn and someone gave me another capsule to swallow. Then a voice said, "Here, let's take off these pajamas and put on this hospital gown." I felt a needle in my buttock, followed by four strong hands moving me onto a trolley. I recall nothing of my trip to the O.R.

My next memory was of awakening in the recovery room. A nurse was leaning over me. I heard her voice through a thick haze. "You're going back to your room now," she said. "The surgery is over." I think I smiled under the thick bandages that wrapped my head. I had been aware of absolutely nothing during the three hours of surgery. My facelift was done. I already felt younger. The relief was enormous. I went back to sleep.

We live in a culture preoccupied with youth. Everything in our society, from television programming and the movies to the news and the specialty magazines, puts heavy emphasis on the young. We are made to feel that the "baby boomers," the "yuppies," and the "18 to 34 market segment" are the fulcrum around which all else in our society revolves, and that our middle-age-and-older population is but one step away from the junk heap, if not the grave. Considering that there are 75,000,000 people in this country who are over the age of forty-five, such emphasis seems incredibly lopsided. Yet, given a choice, where is the person who would not like to look young?

Small wonder that the facelift is growing so rapidly in popularity among men and women over forty (and a few still in their thirties) who want to look youthful longer; because, nowadays, with emphasis on good health and exercise, they *feel* younger. During the first four years of this decade, the number of facelifts performed in the U.S. increased by an astounding 39 percent, and for every one done, there were hundreds, if not thousands, of others that were contemplated by people who are not too happy when they look in the mirror and see what the aging process has done to their looks. Betty Ford's frank discussion on TV and in the press about her own facelift brought this operation out of the closet and into the nation's living rooms. For the first time in history, the wife of a President talked of having a facelift and how the results gave her more than just a pretty face by increasing her confidence and feeling of self-worth.

If you are one of the many people who have contemplated a facelift, don't for a second believe that your thoughts about the possibility of looking better make you an egotist, or that you need to fear voicing your personal interest in cosmetic surgery to those who are close to you. Wanting to look good is as natural as wanting to be thin or healthy. Fortunately, plastic surgery has reached a point where quite a bit can be done for most, if not all, would-be patients. This is not to say that a facelift will make you look as you did in your youth, or that it can turn you into a perennial teen. It can't. But with a realistic approach to such surgery, and a qualified, competent surgeon, the chances are excellent that someone who is a good candidate for a facelift can succeed in camouflaging the aging process to some degree. The exact degree depends upon the physical condition of your face, the thickness and condition of your skin, the presence or absence of facial fat, the relative "age" of your skin, the numbers and types of wrinkles you have, your underlying bone structure, heredity, and hormonal influences.

Let's examine this operation: what is done to your face in a facelift, what results you can expect, the hospitalization, the scars, the anesthesia, the recuperation period, and the psychological aspects. Let's also look at some of the more common myths about facelifts.

What a Facelift Can Do . . . What It Will Not Do

The medical name for a facelift is *rhytidectomy*, and the medical dictionary defines the procedure as the "excision of skin wrinkles, particularly of the face and neck, for cosmetic purposes." This may actually be an overstatement, since a facelift will *not* remove small wrinkles or lines of the upper lip, the cheeks, or forehead. There is another procedure called a *brow and forehead lift* that can elevate your fallen brows as well as improve some of these fine lines and deep frown grooves. And in Chapter 9 I discuss two procedures that improve or eliminate lip wrinkles.

In this chapter I'm going to tell you about the facelift procedure designed to remove redundant skin of the face, particularly of the jawline and the neck, as well as the excess fat located beneath the jaw and chin in the upper neck — above the Adam's apple and beneath the chin. Once again I'd like to point out that calling this procedure a "facelift" is something of a misnomer, since a typical facelift involves lifting the *neck* as well as the face and, occasionally, the brow, forehead, and temple. But since it's common parlance to speak of a "facelift," I'm not going to invent a new name for the procedure.

Each facelift is highly individualized, depending upon the patient's anatomical problems. In some, it is the neck that requires the most attention; in others, it may be the jawline. In general, the best results are achieved by correcting the jawline, lower face, and neck. The results are more dramatic than when surgery is performed on the upper face, temples, and forehead.

As the skin dries and thins out with age, nature and the pull of gravity bestow upon us loose, sagging skin, particularly in the neck, under the chin, and on the cheeks. Most of us develop wrinkles and creases that some people see as a sign of "character" but which others see simply as the telltale marks of old age, something they would just as lief camouflage or get rid of. As time marches on, we also tend to deposit fat along and beneath the jawline and in the upper part of the neck.

What the facelift operation can do is make you look younger and fresher and give your face a more "tidy" appearance. In some people, the change is extraordinary; in others, less so. Much depends on your basic bone structure, with strong bone formation providing the best framework. Since the structure of each face is different, it's difficult to generalize about the results one can expect.

However, of one thing you can be certain: a facelift alone will not change the shape of your face. It will merely restore it, to some degree, to what it was in earlier years. And, unless there is some complication, it will not change your facial expression, either.

I recently did a facelift on a man who had just celebrated his sixtieth birthday. Larry was an interior decorator who had achieved a modest degree of success in his career and who had a wide circle of friends in Saint Louis, his hometown. He had a very appealing personality — witty, outgoing, and urbane. He was a man who liked life and wanted to continue his busy social schedule. He was very realistic about his expectations for the surgery. "I just want to look as good as I feel," he commented. "I want to tighten up these jowls and not look as though my face has been 'lowered' by age." Six months after the operation he told me, "There are times I see myself in the mirror and I can't remember what my face looked like before. It's *me* all right . . . nothing different about the shape of my face, no changes in my features. But that turkey neck is gone, my jowls are firmer, and I think I look *healthier* than I've looked in ages."

The facelift is a complicated and difficult procedure to perform. It almost always calls for extensive correction, more than most people realize, and from the surgeon's point of view, the operation calls for a great deal of judgment and delicacy.

Let's see who are the candidates for this operation.

THE RIGHT CANDIDATES FOR A FACELIFT

Both sexes offer good candidates for facelift surgery, and age is less a factor than the condition of one's skin on the face and neck, the amount of wrinkling that's taken place, and the state of the jaw and neckline. Any mature, psychologically sound person whose aging has left him or her with wrinkles, sagging, or excess fat in the jaw and upper neck region — conditions I've described in the last few pages — can be an excellent candidate for improvement of his or her appearance.

One of the most important considerations in determining whether you are a good candidate for facelift surgery — or *any* type of cosmetic surgery — is the degree to which your expectations for the procedure are *realistic*. A facelift can, as the word implies, *lift* your face, fight the endless downward pull of gravity, and lift your *spirits* at the same time. In some people, it can take years off their appearance; in others, it may create a more youthful, cleaner look around the neck and jaw; in still others, the results may be so subtle that they merely look relaxed and well rested.

So, anyone from thirty-five to seventy-five with any of the facial and skin problems I've been describing, who has the right motivation and is not expecting miracles, is a "right" candidate for a facelift — provided, naturally, that there are no contraindications in the individual's physical health.

You should know that every experienced cosmetic surgeon sees many more people who consider themselves candidates for a facelift than he will operate on. There are a number of reasons for this, including the surgeon's schedule, the would-be patient's schedule or timetable, and an inability to match these two. But, for the most part, the surgeon turns down patients because he doesn't consider them suitable candidates for this procedure. This has nothing to do with the doctor "liking" or "not liking" any individual. Often, it is because a patient wants the operation for the wrong reasons.

The Wrong Candidates for a Facelift

In recent years, facelift surgery has been sought by younger and younger people, many often in their mid- and late thirties. Most plastic surgeons spend a good deal of time trying to convince some of these people — certainly not all of them — that they are not yet candidates for rhytidectomy. Our advice is not always heeded. Patients who are convinced that they need a facelift often "shop" until they find a surgeon who will perform the operation — sometimes with unhappy results if the change is so minimal that the patient cannot detect any change at all.

Other would-be patients, who are in the right age group for this procedure, are not good candidates for it because they have unrealistic expectations about what the surgeon will be able to do to their faces, or because they want the surgery for the wrong reasons. What people say when consulting a surgeon is not always what they mean. Countless patients have said to me, "I'm beginning to look like my mother and I don't like it." What these people are really saying is that they don't want to grow old like their parents — not that they don't like their parents' looks. There is nothing wrong with wanting to look better, or more youthful. What the surgeon must do in one or more consultations with each would-be patient is balance the person's desires and expectations against his own empirical judgment on whether such expectations can be realized through surgery.

A surgeon frequently sees patients whose marriages or other romantic relationships are in trouble. Most often, patients consulting a cosmetic surgeon at such times are women. If the patient seeks a facelift in order to raise her self-esteem or improve her appearance *for her own sake,* that is one thing; if she wants the facelift in order to salvage the relationship, that is a very iffy expectation, and the patient runs the risk of growing angry and bitter when the facelift doesn't help achieve her goals.

Some patients are poor candidates for a facelift from a physical rather than a psychological standpoint. Such patients fall into many categories: people who have developed vertical "furrow" lines between their eyebrows — a condition for which the facelift technique, per se, is unsatisfactory; people who have keloids (a type of benign skin tumor) as a result of previous operations and are, therefore, at greater risk that they will develop them again; people with blood clotting problems, and others. For some such patients, other forms of aesthetic surgery, such as chemabrasion, dermabrasion, brow lifting, or perhaps even collagen injections, would provide better, if temporary, cosmetic results.

The Best Time for a Facelift

There really is no single best time, since people begin to show their age at different times, depending on heredity, hormones, and what kind of exposure their skin has had to sun and wind. But if I had to name a "best" age, I'd say midforties to early fifties. At that age, most people still have sufficient elasticity in their skin, minimal fat deposits, and, particularly if the bone structure is good, with a nice jawline, the expectations for an excellent result can be high.

However, this is not to say that some remarkable results are not possible for women in their sixties and even their seventies if they have managed to keep their youthful appearance through their fifties and also keep their bodies in good shape. At the other end of the spectrum are patients in their forties who have aged prematurely and show it.

Most men who see a doctor about the possibility of a facelift are in their fifties or early sixties. I want to point out that I'm not talking about baggy eyelids here — which are discussed in the chapter on eyelid surgery. Eyelid surgery is frequently performed on men and women in their forties.

Facelifts for Men

While the facelift continues to gain in popularity and accessibility to people at virtually all social levels, in all income brackets, and in all parts of the country, the most stunning increase in the last decade or so has been among men. Fifteen percent of all cosmetic surgery patients today are men. One out of every six who sees a surgeon about a facelift or eyelid surgery is a man. The more sophisticated the community, the higher will be the percentage of men who seek such operations. Two such examples are New York City and Los Angeles. Particularly in the business world, the competition for jobs and promotions tends to favor those who are young or youthful in appearance. Many men in their fifties, not wanting to be passed over for promotions because they work for a company or professional firm where age is viewed as a handicap ("Let's not even consider him for that job . . . he will soon be approaching an age where he can take early retirement" or "Isn't he a bit long in the tooth for a job that requires so much traveling?") — such men have come to recognize that cosmetic surgery can help their careers.

It's a shame that this attitude towards aging men, no matter how competent and productive they are, does exist in the U.S. But we have to live in the real world, and until we can bring about some major attitudinal changes in our culture, I'm all for helping men, as well as women, look younger and better through facial surgery, particularly if it will boost their confidence and help them achieve their personal or career goals.

I clearly remember my first consultation with a handsome gentleman in his midlife — a well-built, well-dressed man. He had salt-and-pepper speckled hair, thick gray sideburns, and clear, sparkling eyes. He walked with a quick step, youthful and athletic. He arrived for the consultation with his wife, a woman of about fifty who was also athletic looking and well groomed. They made a very attractive middle-aged couple.

"Doctor, I have an unusual problem," he began, "and I admit I'm embarrassed to be here. I'm a rabbi, you see, and my congregation is composed of young people who are very liberal in their beliefs. I like to think that I, too, am liberal and progressive. I enjoy being their rabbi, but I am getting to look too old, at least in my own mind, to be representing these young people. Can you do something rather subtle, something that will make me look a bit younger — perhaps even more vigorous — so that when I speak to my congregation I will feel a bit more relaxed and confident?"

Despite his reservations and obvious guilt about having purely elective aesthetic surgery, I performed a facelift to tidy up his sagging neck and jawline, along with a blepharoplasty to remove the tired-looking bags from his eyes. The results were good from his point of view as well as mine. He went back to his flock with renewed confidence. For his particular situation in life, cosmetic surgery offered the right solution to an unusual but realistic problem.

Let's assume you, or someone you know, is a good candidate for a facelift and having found a surgeon you like and have confidence in, you are booked for the operation. Here's what happens before, during and after this type of surgery.

BEFORE THE SURGERY

Photographs

Preoperative medical photographs must be taken by a medical photographer or by your surgeon. If they are to be taken by a medical photographer, your surgeon will most likely provide you with the name of the local person he recommends for this purpose. You will also be given a date by which these photographs must be in your doctor's hands. The photographer will take both front- and side-view shots but, I assure you, you won't want to frame these pictures — they're not meant to please or flatter you; in fact, they're not for you at all. Just as the chest surgeon can't operate in an intelligent way without X rays of the chest, the plastic surgeon can't operate without special medical photographs that show him your face in every detail.

Medication

I tell my patients to take one tablet of Vitamin K every morning for three days prior to surgery, with the last pill taken the day before the operation. This vitamin facilitates blood clotting. You need a prescription for it and it's not to be taken by people with varicose veins or a history of phlebitis or coronary disease.

I also tell my patients to take 1,000 mg. of Vitamin C each day for at least two weeks prior to surgery. The purpose of this is to promote healing.

For two weeks before and after surgery, you should not take aspirin or any aspirin-containing compound (Alka-Seltzer, Anacin, Bufferin, Coricidin, Darvon Compound, Dristan, Excedrin, Fiorinal, Midol, Percodan, etc.). Anacin-3 or Tylenol may be taken.

If you take any of the ibuprofen medications, it is probably a good idea to discontinue them forty-eight hours before surgery, unless they are badly needed for arthritis or other pain.

Avoiding aspirin or any aspirin-containing compound is vitally important, perhaps one of the most important of all preoperative instructions. It has been well established that aspirin slows down blood coagulation by interfering with the ability of the platelets in the blood to agglutinate (adhere to each other). It is this agglutination of platelets that forms the basic substance of a blood clot. There is a normal amount of bleeding of the small blood vessels during surgery, and when the platelets don't agglutinate properly, this bleeding can be excessive. Not only does this interfere with the surgical procedure, but proper healing depends on blood coagulating. This advice about avoiding aspirin or aspirin derivatives or compounds prior to surgery applies equally to prescription drugs and over-the-counter products. Even a single dose can create a problem.

Patients on Premarin and other conjugated estrogens must discontinue it one week prior to surgery. It can be resumed immediately after surgery. Anyone taking Vitamin E should discontinue it two weeks prior to surgery and for two weeks after.

Smoking

It is important that you do not smoke for two weeks prior to surgery. As with the above advice about aspirin, this is not an idle suggestion. Smoking has long been suspected as a major cause of delayed and improper wound healing. We studied the effects of smoking in a series of over 2,000 facelift patients and found that cigarette smoking was the major cause of serious wound-healing complications in a significant percentage of cases. In fact, if you smoke cigarettes and inhale you are at least twelve times more likely than nonsmokers to suffer poor healing of your facelift incisions. Translated, this means prolonged healing periods with a consequent delay in returning to your job or the social scene; and, worse, the final result of the operation can be marred by ugly scars.

If you cannot give up smoking for at least a week, preferably two weeks before surgery, perhaps you are not sufficiently motivated to have the surgery. Presumably, you are going to have an operation to improve your looks and sense of well-being, so it makes little sense for you to jeopardize the result of this procedure by failing to forgo a couple of weeks of smoking. It is equally important to stay away from cigarettes for two days *following* surgery. If you are a smoker, this may be an excellent opportunity to give up the habit altogether.

Where the operation is performed

Facial surgery can be performed either in the hospital or on an outpatient basis in certain accredited clinics or operating suites attached to physicians' offices. (See pp. 35–37.) I prefer to do most facelifts in the hospital, but your surgeon will discuss with you his preference and your options.

Hospital stay

The usual hospital stay is two to three days, one of which is the day prior to the operation.

Admission is usually early in the day so that certain diagnostic tests, such as a chest X ray and an EKG, can be done and laboratory tests completed. You will also be seen by the resident surgeon and, sometimes, by an anesthesiologist. Of course, if you decide to have the operation as an outpatient or ambulatory patient, you will go home the same day that the surgery is performed.

About the Anesthesia

You will be told that you have a choice between a local and a general anesthetic. The decision is up to you, although your surgeon may tell you his preference. A number of factors enter into the decision.

Some surgeons prefer to work with a local; others prefer the general; still others will use either one, depending on the patient's preference. Whichever you choose, a certain amount of local anesthetic will be used, because a dilute solution of adrenaline (which is part of a local anesthetic) is necessarily injected into your face to help control bleeding.

Ordinarily, a local is administered by the surgeon. When a general is used, an anesthesiologist administers it. Experienced anesthesiologists are living encyclopedias of knowledge about physiology and pharmacology (drugs and anesthetics). They are responsible for managing your whole body health during the operation and, in that sense, it seems far safer for any patient who has a medical problem, such as hypertension or diabetes, to choose a general anesthesia and put him- or herself in the hands of a competent anesthesiologist.

General anesthesia for plastic surgery procedures, especially those involving the face, is not the same as the deep anesthesia required to operate on the stomach, lungs, heart, or other organs. Usually, only intravenous drugs, along with oxygen, are given. Gas inhalation is rarely used, and when it is, it's given in very small doses.

Whether you elect a local or a general anesthetic, you will be quite comfortable. If you have a local, you will also be given intravenous sedation to blur your consciousness.

A common myth is that it's necessary for you to be awake so that the surgeon can monitor your facial movements. Actually, facial movements at this stage are completely irrelevant to the procedure, despite what anyone might tell you. Often this argument is advanced to convince a patient that a local is better than a general anesthesia when, in truth, it's because the surgeon, for reasons of his own, prefers a local. Local anesthesia for facial surgery is excellent and, under normal circumstances, works well. If your surgeon expresses a preference when he discusses this subject with you, it's usually a good idea to go along with his preference — unless, of course, your own wishes are strongly in the opposite direction. But don't let anyone convince you that it's safer to have a local anesthesia, or that such a procedure is better because it lets the doctor see your facial movements. Neither is true.

What you will want to consider, however, is the fact that a general anesthesia requires the services of an anesthetist, and this means an additional fee. A local, on the other hand, is usually administered by the surgeon, and it is customary to include this as part of the basic fee. Ordinarily, no additional charge is made.

When You Will Pay Your Bills

You will, in all likelihood, be asked to pay your surgeon's fee in advance of the surgery. The anesthesiologist's bill is usually paid before you leave the hospital or within a week after you go home. If your medical coverage doesn't include a hospital stay for the purpose of cosmetic surgery (and many policies exclude such surgery), you will probably be told to bring a certified check with you to cover the hospital charges. Your surgeon's nurse or secretary will tell you what the practice is in your community.

The Facelift Technique

The face is a bony structure covered by three layers of soft tissue comprised of muscle, fat, and skin. The deepest layer is muscle, which is covered by a layer of loose, fatty tissue. That, in turn, is covered by the skin. What happens in a facelift is that sagging layers of muscle and fat are either removed or repositioned and the skin is then redraped and tightened over the remaining muscle and fat. When muscles are repositioned, this is known as "sculpting." Considerable advances have been made in recent years in the technique of sculpting and, while it is not always done in a facelift, it does make possible some excellent results in patients where the procedure is indicated.

Surgeons are also making extensive use nowadays of fat suctioning to contour the jawline, the neck, and sometimes the face itself. Known as "suction lipectomy," many doctors routinely include this in most facelift procedures. I use suction lipectomy frequently and will describe the technique to you later on.

A facelift operation should take between two and three hours. If eyelid surgery is performed at the same time, add another one to two hours. If the facelift is done in conjunction with a chin implant, the entire procedure will take between three and five hours.

Where the Incisions Are Made

On each side of the head, an incision is made inside the hairline at the temples and is then extended down in front of the ear to the point where the bottom of the ear joins the head. It then circles around under the earlobe, goes up behind the back of the ear, across the bare, hairless area of the skin over the temporal bone behind the ear (the *mastoid*), and enters just above the hairline of the scalp. Shaving the hair that lies in the path of these incisions is unnecessary.

The reason we cut *above* and not *on* the hairline is to enable a postoperative patient to comb his or her hair *over* the incision, thereby hiding it from view at the back of the head. Contrary to anything you may have heard, there are no "secret" or "hidden" incisions known to only a few surgeons. They don't exist. Nor can you perform a facelift operation through incisions located *only* behind the ears.

The modern facelift procedure also involves a small cut just under the chin to provide access so that excessive accumulations of fat under the jawline or in the upper neck can be trimmed away and the *platysma* muscle sculpted, if necessary. The platysma is the muscle in the neck that extends from the face to the clavicle (collarbone).

After the surgeon makes the first incision (he completes one side of the face before doing the other side) the skin is then separated from the fat and muscle that lie underneath — a process known as "undermining." This creates a flap of skin. How much undermining is done depends on how much sagging skin the patient has. It will differ from person to person.

Infinite patience, skill, judgment, artistry, and experience on the part of the surgeon are brought to bear upon the procedure because he is working in areas that have muscles, nerves, and blood vessels. No surgeon can perform the process of undermining without some disturbance of the small nerve endings in the area being worked on. It is this disturbance of the nerve endings that creates the feeling of numbness all patients experience for some months — anywhere from two months to a year — after the surgery. However, in almost all cases, such numbness — which patients frequently describe as "the same feeling you have when the dentist gives you Novocain" — does eventually disappear. After the skin has been undermined, it is rotated and redraped over the new contour. Temporary sutures are put in position and the excess skin is trimmed off. The incision is then sutured.

Operating on a Man

The technique of the facelift performed on a man differs slightly from that performed on a woman. Since the hairline is different, male patients are encouraged to grow their hair a little longer than ordinarily in the weeks prior to surgery, and to keep their sideburns longer, thus growing a big patch of hair around the side of the head and covering the ears. With bald men, a surgeon tries to start the incision just above the ear, so that some of the temple hair can cover the incision.

There is one inconvenient aspect of the facelift in men that women don't have to cope with. During the operation, the beard-bearing skin of the upper neck is pulled back and relocated behind the ear. This means it becomes necessary to shave behind the earlobes — a small price to pay for a more youthful appearance.

In some, but relatively few instances, an incision must be made across the top of the head in order to tighten the forehead or elevate the brows. Such an incision is rare and is impossible in bald men unless they wear a hairpiece.

Fat Suction

I mentioned that fat suction, or suction lipectomy, is often used nowadays during the facelift procedure. You may have heard or read about this process in connection with thigh, buttock, or abdominal reduction. It is a technique that was originally developed in Europe as a method of literally sucking away excessive fat accumulations in certain parts of the body.

Basically, the technique consists of inserting, through a very small cut in the skin, various-sized straws or pipes, known as *cannulas*, and actually sucking out the fatty deposits that lie beneath the skin. Very high vacuum suction is used to accomplish this. The procedure has proven so successful in properly selected patients that it was adapted to facial surgery, where it has been used to remove localized collections of fat from beneath the chin and jawline. The process has also been used to reduce the amount of fat in the lower face itself, as well as in the cheeks.

This technique, which can be likened to sucking a very thick milkshake through a straw, has been adopted by more and more surgeons so that it is now commonplace during many facelift operations. In fact, in some patients where only minor fat accumulations beneath the skin are the problem, rather than loose or sagging skin and muscle, the fat suction technique is sometimes all that's required. It has proven specially effective in facelift patients who are somewhat younger — in their forties — when only limited skin removal is called for. The technique has also proven to be a godsend for very young adults, those in their twenties and thirties, who have inherited fat accumulations in the form of a double chin or similar deformity but who, under no stretch of the imagination, require a facelift procedure. In such young patients, only a tiny stab wound, placed in an inconspicuous spot beneath the chin, is required.

The Platysma Muscle and the SMAS

The most superficial muscle covering the lower face and neck is called the *platysma*. Its neighboring structures are the SMAS — which stands for the *superficial musculoaponeurotic system*. Strange as it may seem, something as technical sounding as this muscle system has become quite familiar to large numbers of people who frequently read articles about cosmetic surgery. In animals, such as the horse or dog, the platysma is a muscle attached to the skin and its purpose is to move the skin in such actions as shaking off water or troublesome insects. However, in man, this muscle is unnecessary — it has remained a remnant without purpose.

At the point in facelift surgery when the incisions have been made around the ears, and a cut has been made under the chin in order to remove or trim fat under the jawline or in the upper part of the neck, a decision must be made by the physician on whether or not surgery should be performed on the platysma and the SMAS.

Thanks to the innovative work of the late Dr. Tord Skoog, an expert Swedish plastic surgeon, as well as others in the U.S.A., Mexico, and elsewhere, we now know how to tighten the deepest layers of the facial tissues so that we can perform what is, in essence, a two-layer facelift, one on the platysma and the SMAS, the other on the skin. The surgeon must have considerable skill and an excellent knowledge of the anatomy because the platysma and SMAS are intimately involved with nerves, blood vessels, and glands of the region, all of which must be preserved and protected during the operation.

The front part of the platysma muscle is often responsible for the vertical, cordlike structures seen in the front of the neck, extending from beneath the chin toward the collarbone. When surgery is performed on this muscle, bands of platysma are tightened or eliminated, so that the person undergoing the surgery, after recovery, has a cleaner, more youthful-looking neck and jawline.

Sculpting the platysma muscle to create a sharp neck-chin angle and to eliminate strong vertical neck folds, with the skin flap draped over the new contour, is a relatively new art being practiced with increasing frequency. After such sculpting, when the skin flap is redraped, it must fill every crevice created in reshaping the muscle. The surgeon's judgment on whether the patient's appearance calls for this procedure and his talents in performing it are why we say that cosmetic surgery calls for a combination of art and science.

Blood Loss

Blood loss is minimal in facelift surgery, and transfusions are extraordinarily rare. In twenty-five years I have transfused only one facelift patient, who had a coagulation abnormality.

If you are contemplating surgery and are greatly afraid of transfusions because of possible AIDS transmission, or because of religious taboos, you might consider having an autotransfusion — that is, a transfusion of your own blood drawn several days before your operation. However, with current techniques for screening blood donors for AIDS, there is no more than one in a hundred thousand chances of contracting the disease through a blood transfusion. Furthermore, with an experienced surgeon, the chances of needing a transfusion during a facelift procedure are less than one in five thousand.

However, there can be some small bleeding during a facelift, known as "oozing," and this can sometimes be troublesome, although not dangerous. The amount of bleeding is determined by many factors that influence the complicated coagulation process. That's why I advise my patients to discontinue all medication containing aspirin for two weeks prior to surgery, since aspirin slows down blood coagulation.

The Scars

If the incisions are properly placed within the hair and in the natural creases around the ear, the resulting scars will be almost, if not 100 percent, invisible. If excessive tension is created during the suturing process, the scars sometimes have a tendency to spread. A stretched scar in the hairline is a nuisance because it will remain a bald area — hair doesn't grow in scar tissue. But bald scars are most apt to occur only after a second or third facelift. Sometimes, but rarely, revision of such wide scars may be helpful and, in severe cases, hair plug transplants offer remedial help.

The scars that occur where the incisions were placed are permanent, but these are more of a nuisance than a tragedy, given the object of the surgery in the first place. The trade-off is worth it. Almost always, the scars are in the natural facial lines so they can be easily camouflaged by makeup or the way the hair is worn. Women who are accustomed to wearing their hair pulled back off the face sometimes like to adopt a new, softer coiffure with some of the hair brushed forward.

The Possibility of Complications

Complications are possible after any kind of surgery — whether it's cosmetic surgery, an appendectomy, a cesarean section, or anything else. Minor, unanticipated complications do sometimes occur as a result of a facelift, but they are uncommon and usually of temporary duration. Elective surgery is a matter of risk vs. benefit. In a facelift, the risk factor is small and the likelihood of benefit is great. But you should be sufficiently informed about the possibility of complications to make an intelligent decision about whether you want to have this surgery.

The most common complication after a facelift is *hematoma*, which is a collection of blood under the skin. This blood accumulation occurs when a small amount of bleeding or oozing continues after the surgery is finished. In about 2 percent to 3 percent of patients with a hematoma, this collection of blood must be removed in the first few hours after surgery, because there is active and continuing bleeding going on beneath the skin. In all other instances of hematoma, it is removed in an office procedure after a week or ten days by *aspirating* it— that is, removing the blood with a needle and a small syringe. In the majority of cases when a small hematoma occurs, however, no treatment at all is required, as the small amount of blood is absorbed into the body over a period of several weeks.

Most patients understand that there will be some amount of bruising and discoloration following a facelift. But the amount of such bruising varies tremendously. Some people look as though they had been in a boxing match. Others appear almost normal. But since we consider the former to be a distinct possibility, I advise my patients to set aside, after surgery, three weeks free of social engagements in order to get over the telltale bruises. If complete facial surgery is being done — that is, a facelift plus eye surgery, plus brow lift, one needs even a bit more time than that, as swelling and bruising are apt to be more noticeable.

One can decrease the chances of even a minor complication by following a few simple precautions during the immediate postoperative period. During the first twenty-four hours after surgery, a quiet, calm atmosphere is encouraged, since it is during this period that complications can occur. For perhaps forty-eight hours after surgery, I suggest a liquid and soft food diet. I also tell my patients to avoid keeping their head down for long periods of time as the force of gravity will increase the swelling. If it's necessary to bend, do so at the knees. It is also important that a post-op facelift patient sleep on his or her back, with the head elevated on one or two pillows, for ten days following the surgery.

Also: no strenuous activities such as exercise, jogging, sports, dancing, or heavy housecleaning are permitted for three weeks following surgery. And it is probably not a good idea to have sex during the first week after surgery. Alcoholic beverages should be avoided for at least a week following surgery, as alcohol tends to increase swelling and the chance of bleeding. Saunas and steam baths should be avoided for a month, and flying is not recommended until all the sutures have been removed.

Of course, fate and nature sometimes combine to thwart even our best attempts to prevent complications. Other complications, such as nerve paralysis, infection, skin ulceration, scar overgrowth, pigment irregularities, and burst capillaries can also occur, but they are quite uncommon.

Nerve Injury During Surgery

The nerve supply to the face is rich and complicated, with considerable overlapping of nerves, which in different people are not always located in the same anatomical position. One of the calculated risks one takes when having facial surgery is the risk of some complication due to the injury or cutting of a nerve. The nerves which supply sensation, the sensory nerves, are always cut when an incision is made. There is no way around this. Consequently, sensation over much of the facial, ear, and neck skin may be diminished or absent entirely for several weeks or even a few months after the operation. This occurs especially around the ears and sometimes includes part of the ears themselves. Occasionally, very small areas of numbness persist permanently.

In the modern, extended facelift operation, it is very important for the doctor to avoid damaging the nerves that supply facial expression and to know the "safe" limit when undermining the facial tissue. It is particularly important to exercise great care at the precise point over the jawbone where a small nerve emerges from beneath the platysma muscle to supply the muscles of the lower lip and the mouth. During the undermining process, this nerve, or branches of it, are sometimes stretched, bruised, or otherwise injured, resulting in a weakness of the lip that can persist for weeks, sometimes for several months. Fortunately, in almost all instances, this disappears. Should the nerve be cut in half during the surgery, return of function in the lip muscles is unlikely. Injury to nerves that control the muscles of the cheeks, eyelids, brow, and forehead can also occur, but this is exceedingly rare. A permanent injury is so rare that you really shouldn't be at all concerned about it if you have selected a qualified, competent surgeon.

An uncomfortable feeling of tightness across the neck is not unusual following surgical tightening of the platysma muscle, but this gradually eases up during the first few months after the operation. Again, this is exceedingly rare, but should the platysma muscle be cut during surgery, a prominent Adam's apple can develop in those few patients who have an anatomical predisposition to it.

Anything that interferes with normal blood flow can cause "skin death." After a facelift, a loss of blood supply can sometimes cause localized skin sloughing — that is, a thick scab of dead skin. When this occurs, it is most often the skin just behind the ears that is involved.

While this cannot properly be called a "complication," I do want to mention something referred to as a "pulled look." This is a distinctly unnatural look that can result from excessive surgery. The reaction to Betty Ford's operation after the public recovered from the shock of learning that a President's wife had admitted publicly to having had a facelift, was either that she looked "gorgeous" or that she looked "too tight." What they meant by the latter was that her face, particularly the lower half, had a "pulled look." Many facelifts do, indeed, look "too tight" or "pulled" for weeks, or maybe six months, after surgery, eventually loosening up and regaining a normal appearance. However, when it occurs after many repeat operations, it can be permanent.

AFTER THE SURGERY

Bandages

Bandages are applied to the head and neck after a facelift. These are removed forty-eight hours after surgery. Although bandages will not prevent bruising and swelling, they help minimize them. Bandages are applied for another reason. The operated area should be kept as immobile as possible for the first two days after surgery, and bandages help do that. For the same reason, I urge my patients to keep telephone calls and visits to a minimum during this period.

Pain

Postoperative pain is rare. Whatever discomfort you may experience is mild, short-lived, and easily handled with routine medication.

Removal of stitches

After a facelift, some stitches in front of the ears are removed on the sixth or seventh day. In most instances, the remaining stitches are removed by the tenth day. The removal of stitches is quick and uncomplicated, as well as painless. Stitches are usually removed by a nurse or assistant.

Makeup

Facial makeup can usually be applied by the tenth day. If bruises are still present, you may want to use some type of covering cream. At the end of each day, it is important to remove all makeup thoroughly, using an upward motion. Oiled eyepads are recommended for the removal of eye makeup.

Getting your hair done

On the fourth day following surgery, you may comb your hair by using warm water and a large-toothed comb. Your first shampoo is possible on the sixth day following surgery. Rollers may be used, but loosely. If your hair is blown dry, it should be with a dryer turned to "Warm," not "Hot." If you sit under a dryer, turn the control to "Comfort Zone." Tinting and coloring may usually be done about three weeks after the operation.

Postoperative depression

Many patients go through a temporary period of slight emotional depression immediately following surgery. This is quite normal and should not alarm you. It is not easy to look bruised and swollen and be happy about it — particularly since your objective in the first place was to improve your appearance. Rest assured that this period will pass quickly.

Appearing in public

After the swelling and bruising disappear, you may go through a period when you look strange even to yourself. The length of this period varies patient-to-patient and also depends upon whether you had a simple facelift or combined it with a second cosmetic surgical procedure. I tell my patients to set aside three weeks, postoperatively, when they may want to see only close friends. At the end of that period, you should be ready to go back to work, although this depends upon whether you want to be secretive about the surgery you had.

When patients tell me they prefer to hide the fact that they've had a facelift, I encourage them to change their hairstyle and even their makeup after surgery — sometimes to change their hair color. This way, if friends detect some difference in appearance, it can be attributed to the changes in hairstyle or makeup. Men do well to grow a moustache or beard if they wish to camouflage the facelift results temporarily. Men patients, and some women as well, are unaccustomed to using makeup and don't care to do so after surgery. Fortunately, the facelift scars are so well hidden that this is not a problem.

The Months Following Surgery

Your facelift will "settle" during the first few months after surgery. Some of the redundant skin folds may return — this is not uncommon. Most patients are distressed when they see the return of small defects that were not there immediately after the operation. In fact, six months after surgery, patients frequently complain that they don't look quite as good as they did right after the operation. Few people are spared this passing disappointment. However, the good news is that, after about six months of settling, the result stabilizes for several years, subject to the natural aging process. In a few patients, minor corrections are required after the initial surgery. If this should happen to you, don't feel singled out for an unhappy result, or that the surgeon didn't do his best work. It is not related to the surgeon's expertise, or to anything you did or failed to do during the recuperation period. It is due to the fact that cosmetic surgery is as much an art as a science, and even the greatest artists of all time had, occasionally, to rework a section of a painting. And living flesh is even less predictable than an inanimate painting.

When some minor adjustment is indicated and a second surgical procedure is performed, it does not usually take place until six to twelve months after the initial operation. It is done, almost always, on an ambulatory basis — in and out of the clinic or hospital on the same day. In the case of such small corrective work, many surgeons will not charge a second fee. However, the patient does have to pay a hospital or ambulatory facility bill.

One patient who had developed a small hematoma after her facelift was initially troubled by the very small, almost minuscule bulge that remained even after the hematoma had subsided. She was told that in about six months the surgeon would perform a minor procedure in his office to remove it. She agreed. But when

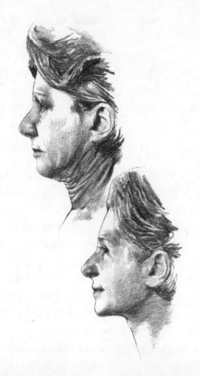
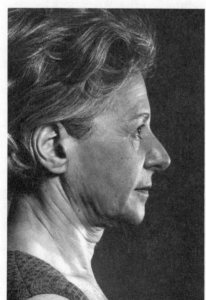
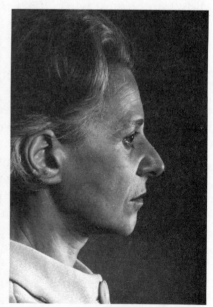

Results of facelift surgery that eliminated loose skin on face and neck.

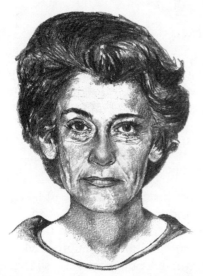
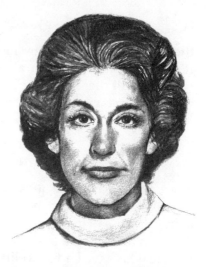

The rejuvenating effect of a facelift combined with eyelid surgery is clearly seen in this before-and-after comparison of an attractive woman in her forties. Strong, well-defined bone structure made her an excellent candidate for the facelift procedure.

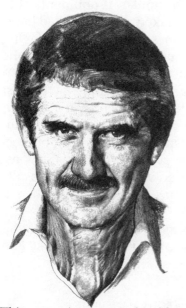
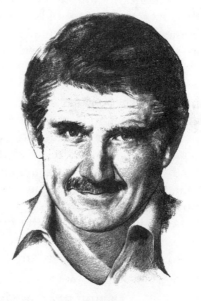

This attractive man in his fifties achieved a clean jawline and a more youthful appearance after facelift surgery removed sagging tissue of his neck and lower face.

the six months were over she said, "I don't notice it any more. It's blended into the natural look of my face and I'm quite comfortable with that look. I never wanted to look *perfect*. . . . I only wanted some improvement in my appearance, and I got it. Let's leave things as they are."

Looking to the Future

Every patient asks the question "How long will my facelift last?" This is hard to predict because of individual differences in the aging process. The modern extended facelift is expected to last for eight to ten years under normal circumstances of aging. Most people who have had a facelift eventually come back for a second lift — a clear indication that they were happy with the first one. They want to continue to camouflage the aging process.

The results of a second facelift are usually as good as, or better than, the first one and will probably last longer. This may be due to the fact there is already a small layer of scar tissue just under the skin and this provides a scaffold on which to build. The second operation is usually quite similar, if not identical to the first one, in terms of how much is taken away or pulled back. Someone who has several facelifts does run the risk of having a "stretched" facial expression, because by that time in life the skin will very likely have lost its elasticity.

But enough about "complications." Most people — the vast majority, I would say — are very happy to have had a facelift, and their reactions most often are decidedly positive. It is indicative of their satisfaction that so many of these people recommend friends and relatives to their surgeons for consultations. It's because most people are so pleased with the surgical results that this type of cosmetic surgery has grown so markedly in popularity.

Of course, there *are* the myths and misconceptions that always spring up concerning any type of cosmetic surgery — and this is as good a time as any to debunk them for you.

Debunking the Myths about Facelifts

Although it is often heralded in some of the women's magazines, there is no such thing as a "mini-lift." That expression, sometimes referred to as a "little tuck," came about in this way. R. Passot, a Frenchman, designed the first facelift operation in the early part of this century. What he did was remove a small piece of skin, cut away from in front of the ears, after which the face was pulled up. This is, in essence, what people mean when they speak of "mini-lifts."

However, the result of Passot's procedure, which used to be very popular in Europe, mostly performed by surgeons untrained in the true art of facelift surgery, was only temporary, lasting anywhere from a few weeks to a few months, at best. Such "nips and tucks" are sometimes effective in making small corrections after a proper facelift operation. Unfortunately, repeated "nips and tucks" will not maintain a facelift for very long.

Here's another one that falls in the myth department. Beware of any advertisement that reads, "Do your facelift on a lunch hour and be back at work the same afternoon." Don't believe it. There's no such thing. While it's technically possible, I'd feel mighty sorry for the patient and very pessimistic about the long-term results of that operation.

What a skilled surgeon can do in a facelift procedure takes time, patience, judgment, and skill. And the procedure calls for a proper, aseptic operating facility, with the right operating room equipment and personnel; anesthesia; time spent in a recovery room; and a convalescent period of days or weeks, depending on how extensive the operation was and how the patient handled it. I would urge you to be very skeptical in evaluating promises of "quick cures."

There is yet another myth, more a misconception, which tells you that skin damaged by a lifetime of exposure to sun and wind can be restored by surgery. Once the skin's elasticity is gone, nothing can bring it back. While a facelift can tighten loose skin, elasticity, once gone, is gone forever.

And then there is the myth that has to do with nonsurgical procedures which claim to accomplish the same thing as a facelift operation through the use of creams, lotions, skin tighteners, masks and mousses, or other cosmetic products. While some of these products do have merit as lubricants and moisturizers, they will not eradicate wrinkles or lift a sagging jowl. This is not to say that some such items will not make your skin feel better or softer to the touch. But accomplish the same as a facelift? They simply can't do it.

Do not be taken in by advertisements that claim a facelift can be accomplished with acupuncture, either. Acupuncture may have many bona fide medical uses, but they do not include the ability to eradicate a sagging jawline or what we refer to medically as a "turkey" neck. Those who claim otherwise are either completely unscrupulous or are basing their claims on the subjective reports of patients who have provided information that is not altogether accurate. No one has produced any creditable documentation that acupuncture can have a beneficial effect on the anatomical deformities of the aging face. Keep in mind that pre- and postoperative photographs can be doctored in the darkroom. Discount any claims about acupuncture being a substitute for a surgical facelift.

Another claim frequently heard these days is that a facelift can be effectively and simply performed with a laser. Lasers are wonderful medical instruments. They have many uses in medicine and can literally perform miracles in such things as eye surgery. But, as of this writing, lasers have not been developed to the point where they are of any use in a facelift. A giant hoax was recently exposed where unscrupulous operators were claiming to achieve facelift results without surgery, merely by passing a "laser light" over the skin. The light proved to be a simple fluorescent light without any medical benefit whatsoever. Be careful of such propaganda. Always ask a qualified physician about such reports. We'd all like to have the benefits of surgery without undergoing the discomfort of an operative procedure but, as yet, there simply is no substitute for it in facelifting.

More than Just a Pretty Face . . .

For every person who believes in one of the myths I've just recounted, there are hundreds of others who want cosmetic surgery, consult with an experienced and accredited surgeon, undergo the operation, and come away simply delighted with the results. For Mary, a fifty-four-year-old successful, energetic lady who had come north from Atlanta after college and pursued a highly rewarding career in public relations and advertising in New York

City, a facelift meant much more than just a pretty face . . . much more.

I remember the very day when I first gave serious consideration to having a facelift. The advertising business is a grueling one and I've worked in it like a demon for more than twenty years, first in the advertising department of Rich's Department Store in Atlanta, and then in some of the better New York agencies. Not only am I the highest ranking woman executive in my present company, but I think I must be the oldest one in a position of responsibility. Generally, it's a young people's business; they want to get them young and train them in the company culture.

Well, it had been a particularly taxing day, deadlines to meet, the phone never stopped ringing, and in the afternoon we got the bad news that a new piece of business we had solicited had been assigned to another up-and-coming agency. Our CEO called a meeting of the group that had made the new business presentation, including me, and said among other things that ". . . maybe we should put a whole new team against our new business effort, maybe put some of our hot Young Turks on it, the kids who could really relate to the M.B.A.s on the client side."

I went home feeling rotten, and when I looked in the bathroom mirror, what I saw was a fifty-four-year-old woman who was, all of a sudden, looking old and haggard. People had always taken me for much younger than my age . . . at fifty I could easily have passed for forty or forty-two. I didn't feel burnt out . . . my health was excellent and my energy level was, to quote my twenty-three-year-old secretary, "breathtaking." I knew that I accomplished more in a single day than any two of the younger "Turks" in my company. I wondered if the CEO had been referring to me or others in the group around my age, when he said he wanted a younger team put in place.

That was the day I decided to see a doctor about a facelift, and I can't tell you what it's done for me. The truth is, I was never really threatened in my job; but deep inside I had this nagging feeling that perhaps the firm's management felt that I had had it. Had I been terminated, I would have known it was not for the quality of my work, which was and continues to be excellent. It would have been strictly because I was working with people on the client side who were often younger than I. Many of these young men don't like to work with so-called older women.

It isn't that anything has changed externally since the facelift. My job is the same; so are the people around me. But when I look in the mirror I see a woman who's youthful, with a neat, tidy chinline and a good neck and very few wrinkles other than a couple of smile lines near my eyes. I have a much more positive image of myself and a general feeling of psychological well-being. I feel that I've made a new beginning, that I can hack it with any of them, and that age is no longer a negative factor in my career. If anything, the youthful appearance, combined with my years of experience, give me a unique advantage. Knowing all this has actually changed the expression on my face to one of cheerfulness and pleasure. I owe a lot to modern surgery.

" 'Tis not a lip, or eye, we beauty call,
But the joint force and full result of all."

— ALEXANDER POPE,
An Essay on Criticism

Improving the Chin and the Jaw | 6

I WAS A LATE BLOOMER. *I never thought much about my looks until I was in high school. Then boys became our big preoccupation and though I was far from unpopular, I began to feel envious of my friends who were pretty. I felt that my nose was too big for my face, which seemed otherwise OK to me, particularly since I never had acne. I knew I had a small chin, but that never struck me as part of my problem. I began to read articles in different magazines about cosmetic surgery that had been done on teenagers and I asked my parents (they both have nice noses) if the nose I had inherited from my grandmother couldn't be made smaller.*

At first my parents said I was pretty enough and that, as I grew older, my face would mature and my nose would fit it better. But my grandmother, who had always hated her own nose, became my ally in convincing my folks that I should have plastic surgery on my nose when I graduated from high school. She even offered to pay for it. My father agreed reluctantly, but my mother soon became a real convert to the idea.

The amazing thing is that none of us mentioned my chin, or even thought about it, as far as I can recall. Though it was definitely receded, it never occurred to me that a bigger chin would give me a better profile look — I always thought it was the prominent nose that determined my weak profile. I couldn't have been more surprised when the doctor sug-

gested that I should also have a small chin implant done when he did my nose. In fact, I had never heard of a chin implant, although since I had it done I've heard about it a lot.

I really, truly am happy with my face now. It worked out the way I wanted it. But I couldn't tell you which helped more, the change in my chin or the change in my nose. Maybe it was the combination. Anyway, I think I have a nice look, all around, and it's definitely a good profile. I can't complain. Any way you look at it, I have a much better face than I was born with.

The artist looking at the human face divides its structure into anatomical thirds: the upper face, or brow area; the midface, which includes the nose and the underlying bone structure or upper jaw (the *maxilla*); and the lower face, which contains the lower jawbone (the *mandible*) and the chin. For these proportions to be aesthetically pleasing and for a person to have an attractive profile, these anatomical landmarks of chin, nose, and forehead should be in reasonable harmony. Classical proportions suggest equal thirds.

Even people concerned with improving their looks, people who study their face from every angle, rarely think in terms of aesthetically pleasing proportions of chin, nose, and forehead. While they pay a great deal of attention to the size and shape of their nose, to the number of wrinkles they develop, and to the tissues around the eyes, they tend to overlook and underestimate the importance of the shape, size, and thrust of the chin as a determining factor in the overall appearance of the face.

Despite the fact that a receding chin is a most common facial characteristic, it is amazing how many people never mention this anatomical imperfection when visiting a plastic surgeon to discuss a nose operation or a facelift. Even less frequently are they aware that this problem can be corrected with a procedure that can be performed at the same time as the rhinoplasty (nose operation) or facelift. In fact, about 15 percent of the people who can be helped by nasal plastic surgery are also good candidates for chin augmentation.

As I said, many people seeking other types of facial surgery are not aware that their chin is out of balance with the rest of the face until it's pointed out to them or until they see medical photographs of their profile that graphically demonstrate it. The profile, in particular, is strongly influenced by the jawline and especially by the projection of the chin. Even a well-shaped or reshaped nose that has excellent lines may not do much to improve one's looks, overall, without a properly proportioned chin. In either a facelift or a rhinoplasty, a corrective procedure on the chin can be every bit as important as the surgery that brought a patient to a surgeon in the first place. Personally, I think it's unwise for a surgeon to suggest an operation to correct a defect of which a person is unaware. But chin augmentation, in my opinion, is an exception to this rule of thumb.

Two Groups of Jaw Surgery

The basic look and contour of one's face is, of course, genetically determined; but the plastic surgeon can, when called for, intervene where hereditary forces have created a facial imbalance or disharmony.

Since the jaw stops growing at about the age of sixteen, any time after that can be considered a proper time for jaw surgery. However, if the procedure is to involve surgery on the jawbone, most surgeons will recommend waiting until the late teens or until the patient is in her or his twenties.

Corrective procedures performed on the jaw fall into two categories: those that *enlarge* or *augment* the small or recessive chin; and those that *reposition* or *decrease the size* of an overly protruding jaw. A receding chin can often be corrected with an implant; decreasing the size of the jaw requires surgery on the bone itself. Most cosmetic surgery on the jaw is of the former type. In this chapter I will tell you about those mild or moderate deviations of the jaw's size, shape, and projection that are of common concern, and about the possibilities for altering an underdeveloped or overdeveloped jaw.

Jaw surgery is not a recent development, although the techniques used in such operations have advanced greatly in recent years. In the late nineteenth century, President Grover Cleveland suffered cancer of the upper jaw and, for aesthetic reasons, a leading surgeon removed his entire upper jaw and replaced it with one made of vulcanized rubber. The cancer did not recur and Cleveland was able to bite, chew, and speak without apparent difficulty.

Nowadays, surgery on both the upper and lower jaws is commonplace. Unlike other cosmetic procedures, diagnosis of a jaw problem — except where a simple chin augmentation is indicated — requires more than an office examination. Careful preoperative diagnosis and planning will call for everything from CAT scans and special X rays to dental models. Often, these are cases where the need for jaw surgery stems less from cosmetic concerns and more from the fact that a person is suffering some functional impairment.

When one or both jaws grow too much or too little, the result can be improper biting, chewing, speaking, even breathing. In such cases, patients tend to consult an oral surgeon because the cosmetic aspect of their condition bothers them less than the impairment in function. However, both dental surgeons and plastic surgeons perform operations in which the jaw is reshaped or repositioned. Sometimes, to correct a complicated jaw and teeth problem, a plastic surgeon will work in concert with an oral surgeon.

Treating the Recessed Chin

The most common operation on the lower part of the face is chin augmentation, which increases the size and projection of the chin and, in so doing, aesthetically improves the harmonious relationship between the two lower thirds of the face. This procedure, known as *mentoplasty*, can be performed surgically by two different techniques, one a bit more complicated than the other. In just about every case, this operation does an excellent job of improving a person's profile; and patient satisfaction with the results runs high.

The Techniques

The simpler, more commonly used method involves a chin implant. It is effective in augmenting the slightly to moderately recessed chin. An incision is made in the small natural crease just under the chin; or, as an alternate method, inside the mouth through the "gutter" at the bottom of the lip where it meets the jawbone. Both of these incisions are very small and, in terms of visibility, quite inconsequential. Because the external cut located under the chin is in a spot where hardly anyone would notice it, the small scar is nothing at all to be concerned about. And since so many of us, as infants or children, fell out of a crib, a sleigh, or from a bicycle, a small under-the-chin scar is commonplace.

Through either of those incisions, the surgeon creates a pocket on the front surface of the jaw, in the chin area. The size of the pocket is determined by the size and shape of the implant he will use. Usually made of silicone rubber, the implant is carved and fitted onto the front surface of the mandible, just at the point of the chin and along the side of the jaw. There is considerable variance in the size and shape of this implant, depending on what the surgeon deems necessary to achieve a pleasing result. Nestled in its pocket, the implant is fixed there by sutures in the skin or inside the mouth.

A chin implant can easily be done in the same surgical session as a rhinoplasty or facelift. Many surgeons prefer to do the chin surgery first, because its results can give them better perspective in performing either the rhinoplasty or the facelift.

The second method of augmenting the chin so that its point projects forward involves cutting through the bone of the mandible itself. This cut is made in a horizontal plane above the lower edge of the bone along the chinline. The chin segment that has been cut free from the main body of the mandible is then slid forward in a manner similar to pulling open a drawer. This bone segment is then wired into position, the wires fixing the edges of the cut bone to each other to stabilize the fracture. However, the *jaws* are not wired shut, so there is little interference with such functions as talking or chewing.

This technique is known as the "sliding horizontal osteotomy" or "bone cut" and is the method of choice of many surgeons. The advantage of this method is that the appearance of the chin is improved by altering the bony architecture of the jawbone itself without the need for an implant. Most surgeons make their choice between the two chin augmentation procedures based on their evaluation of the patient's condition.

In extreme degrees of chin deformity, the jaw is not only cut and repositioned but bone grafts, and sometimes artificial implants, are also used to augment the size and thrust of the chin.

Hospitalization and Anesthesia

As with most other cosmetic surgery, a simple chin implant can be done either on an ambulatory, outpatient basis or in a hospital. When surgery on the bone is required to reposition the jaw, hospitalization for a few days is usually required.

Chin augmentation is usually done under local anesthesia, combined with a light sedative. However, if it is being done in conjunction with a facelift or nose operation, which is usually the case, and the patient and doctor have agreed on a general anesthesia, the chin procedure is also performed under the general.

BEFORE THE SURGERY

Photographs — Preoperative medical photographs must be taken by a medical photographer or by your surgeon. The photographer will take both front- and side-view shots so that your surgeon will have a precise picture of your profile, as well as a full front view. If your chin augmentation is to be performed in conjunction with another cosmetic procedure, such as nasal surgery or a facelift, all the necessary pictures will be taken in the same photographic session.

Medication — I prescribe for my patients one tablet of Vitamin K every morning for three days prior to surgery, the last pill to be taken the day before the operation. This vitamin promotes blood clotting. It's a prescription drug and is not to be taken by anyone with varicose veins, phlebitis, or coronary disease. Whether you undergo a simple chin operation or have that procedure in conjunction with another one, the amount of Vitamin K prescribed will be the same.

I also tell my patients to take 1,000 mg. of Vitamin C each day for two weeks prior to surgery to promote healing.

You should not take aspirin or any drug containing aspirin for two weeks before and after surgery. This would include Alka-Seltzer, Anacin, Bufferin, Coricidin, Darvon Compound, Dristan, Excedrin, Fiorinal, Midol, and Percodan. Aspirin slows down blood coagulation by interfering with the ability of the platelets in the blood to adhere to each other. A small amount of normal bleeding during surgery can become excessive if the blood fails to clot properly. Anacin-3 and Tylenol are permissible because they do not contain aspirin. If you take any of the ibuprofen medications, it is probably a good idea to discontinue them forty-eight hours before surgery, unless they are badly needed for arthritis or other pain.

AFTER THE SURGERY

Bandages

After the augmentation procedure, the chin is strapped with special tape for three or four days to help hold the implant in position and to exert pressure on the skin over the implant in order to prevent bleeding. When the tape strapping is removed, a very small bandage is applied to the external incision, if the surgery was performed through an external pocket.

Medication

Postsurgically, some physicians prescribe a broad-spectrum antibiotic (one that is effective against a wide range of bacteria) as a preventive measure against infection.

If the incision was made inside the mouth, it's a good idea to use a weak

	peroxide solution as a mouthwash for a week or so, in order to keep the incision line clean.
Diet	To avoid undue movement of the jaw, a liquid or soft diet is prescribed for several days after surgery. After that, there are no dietary restrictions.
Pain	With a simple chin augmentation, there is rarely any significant pain, but the pressure of the implant can be quite uncomfortable for a few days. If combined with a facelift or rhinoplasty, the chin area can be more uncomfortable than the areas operated on for either of the other procedures. Some patients complain of a feeling of "fullness" of the chin, and this can last for several weeks. I believe this is caused by the presence of the silicone mass, to which they are unaccustomed. Gradually, the swelling subsides and so does the discomfort. When direct surgery on the jaw has been done, more discomfort can be felt, although it is nothing that mild pain medication cannot relieve in most patients.

Technique for Treating the Protruding Jaw

The opposite of a small, recessed chin is the large protruding jaw. It is a facial imperfection often accompanied by malocclusion of the teeth — the lower teeth project forward of the uppers, creating the opposite of an overbite. This type of facial imperfection is referred to as the "Hapsburg jaw," since it was a genetic trait of that European dynasty. It is also sometimes called a "hammer jaw."

The medical name for the condition is *prognathia*. In extreme cases, where teeth are badly out of alignment, surgery is used to reposition the lower jaw, enabling the teeth to meet. At the same time, the contour of the face is also markedly improved.

Where the protrusion of the lower jaw is slight, the procedure usually calls for scraping away a part of the bone through an incision made inside the mouth. The scar is not troublesome and is located in the "gutter" behind the lower lip, where it meets the jaw.

In contrast to the relative simplicity of correcting a recessed chin, repair of a protruding jaw is a major surgical procedure. It is performed in the hospital, under general anesthesia, and it takes anywhere from two to four hours.

Since this anatomical defect is usually associated with a severe malocclusion of the teeth, the lower jaw has to be reconstructed, which calls for cutting through the bone and pushing the lower jaw backwards into a more normal relationship with the upper jaw. In such cases, it is most important to bring the teeth into proper alignment. For this reason, a plastic surgeon often teams up with an orthodontist, an oral surgeon, and a dentist to achieve optimum results.

BEFORE THE SURGERY

Photographs

When you are scheduled for surgery, you will also be scheduled for preoperative photographs to be taken by a medical photographer or by the doctor himself. These photographs are essential so that the surgeon can carefully evaluate your facial structure and help in the preoperative planning of what he will do. They will not be pictures suitable for framing, since they will not be taken to flatter you but to show, in detail, the problem that brought you to a surgeon's office.

Medication

When patients are scheduled for this operation, I prescribe 1,000 mg. of Vitamin C each day for two weeks before the operation. This helps in the healing process.

I also instruct my patients to avoid taking aspirin or any aspirin-containing drugs for two weeks prior to, and for two weeks after surgery. Aspirin slows down blood coagulation because it interferes with the ability of the blood platelets to clot. When clotting is interfered with, excessive bleeding can occur and hinder the healing process.

Aspirin-containing drugs or compounds that you should avoid during this period include Bufferin, Anacin, Alka-Seltzer, Excedrin, Fiorinal, Midol, Darvon Compound, Dristan, Coricidin, and Percodan. Anacin-3 or Tylenol may be taken. If you take any of the ibuprofen medications, it is probably a good idea to discontinue them forty-eight hours before surgery, unless they are badly needed for arthritis or other pain. If you are on any prescription drugs, check with the prescribing doctor or with your cosmetic surgeon on whether such drugs contain aspirin or aspirin derivatives. Bear in mind that even a single dose can create a problem.

Hospital stay

The hospital stay for this operation is longer than for most other facial surgery — perhaps as long as a week, with another week of at-home convalescence.

Paying your bills

As with all cosmetic procedures, your surgeon's fee will be payable in advance of the operation. Since this surgery is performed under a general anesthesia, it will be necessary for you to pay also for the services of an anesthesiologist, whose bill will probably be given to you before you leave the hospital. If this surgery is not covered by your insurance (most cosmetic surgery is *not* reimbursable), you will also be responsible for your hospital charges. For such surgery, most hospitals ask that you pay your bill when you are admitted. Some hospitals ask for a certified check. If it can be demonstrated that your surgery was necessitated by a malfunctioning jaw and not for cosmetic reasons, it may be possible for you to obtain reimbursement from your insurance company. This is something you will want to look into.

AFTER THE SURGERY

Bandages After the operation, a firm pressure bandage is applied to the face and left in place for two days. This helps to keep down the swelling which usually occurs. Because it will be approximately six to eight weeks after surgery before your jaw will be allowed to function, your teeth will be wired together to avoid premature jaw movement. Despite this, many types of food can be consumed if they are liquefied in a blender.

Numbness The jaw may remain numb for many weeks after surgery; sometimes for several months. However, with rare exception, this will gradually go away and sensitivity will return.

POSSIBILITY OF COMPLICATIONS

As with any surgery, complications are always a possibility but in the case of chin augmentation or reduction, they are unlikely. Infection can occur after any operation, but even this is uncommon. Should it occur, it requires prompt treatment with antibiotics.

Postoperative bleeding after either chin augmentation or reduction hardly ever poses a problem.

After chin augmentation, temporary loss of sensitivity in the area of the implant and lower lip is a distinct possibility — I might even say a likelihood. This can last weeks, sometimes months, depending on the patient. Such sensation problems are due to pressure on, or injury to, a small nerve that emerges from the mandible on either side, very near where the lower canine teeth are located. This nerve supplies sensation to the entire lower lip and chin region, and it is easy to shock the nerve during surgery because of the pressure put on it by the implant. Where it exits from the bone, the nerve can also be stretched at the time of the dissection of the pocket. Fortunately, almost all of these sensation losses are temporary. While a permanent loss of sensation (*anesthesia*) of a portion of the lower lip and chin can occur, this is exceedingly rare. Should you experience any sensation loss after surgery, you will want to mention it to your surgeon during your postoperative checkup.

As I mentioned previously, numbness after an operation to correct a protruding jaw is also a distinct possibility, but this is not really a "complication," since it is anticipated.

The plastic implants used in chin augmentation do not elicit an allergic reaction from the body. However, it is possible for them to be expelled (*extruded*). Almost always, this occurs because the pocket that holds them is too tight; or an infection has developed around the implant. In addition, the human body can also be ornery at times, as well as unpredictable, deciding all of a sudden that it wants to reject a foreign body. Even the best placed implant can shift its position or form a pressure point that calls for its removal or replacement. Replacement of an implant, if necessary, is a minor procedure that can be done on an ambulatory basis in less than an hour.

Cosmetic Surgery on the Upper Jaw

It is also possible for the maxilla, the upper jaw, to be too long, too small, or subject to problems that stem from poor positioning or development. A recessed upper jaw can result in a flattened midface region.

Because of the recent advances in *craniofacial* surgery (surgery of the skull and face), which has become a new subspecialty of plastic surgery, the maxilla can also be reshaped and resculpted. For example, the upper jawbone can be cut through its horizontal

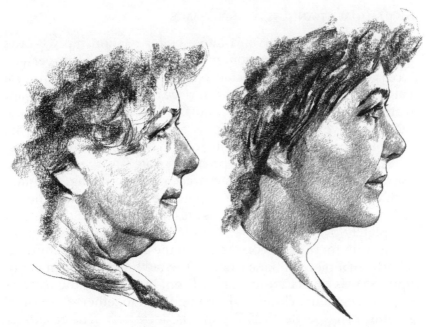

Achieving a clean neck- and jawline sometimes calls for surgical removal of fat accumulations and tightening of jaw muscles.

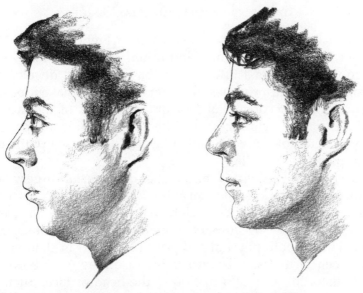

This man's profile was improved by augmentation of his chin with an implant, along with removal of excess fat.

length and brought forward into a better relationship with the lower jaw. In the more common, minor degree of upper jaw recession, a surgeon can achieve more forward projection for a patient by building up the front surface of the bone with implant materials such as silicone or Proplast. Through incisions in the mouth or eyelids, these implants are placed directly over the deficient bone, providing substance and bulk to the cheekbones.

Another, quite common problem related to the upper jaw, the "long face syndrome," is characterized by a long, thin face with excessive exposure of the upper teeth and gums — the so-called gummy smile. The soft tissues are simply too short to fit completely over a bone that's too long. Treatment of this syndrome calls for the surgeon to shorten the upper jaw by removing a horizontal piece of bone from it. The teeth-bearing segment of upper jaw is displaced upwards. Then, by drawing the remaining jaw segments closer and joining them together, the visible amount of upper teeth and gums is decreased. The results of this procedure are quite remarkable. The elongated face is shortened, and the smile that previously exposed the teeth and gums now appears natural and pleasant.

Advances in Craniofacial Surgery

Craniofacial surgery was pioneered by a Frenchman, Dr. Paul Tessier, and, thanks to him and others who have followed in his footsteps, the last fifteen years have seen the development of some radical approaches to surgery that now make it possible to correct major congenital or acquired defects of the face and skull. The new techniques give the surgeon wide access to the bony skeleton of the skull so that he can literally sculpt the bone as he pleases.

Each week I see virtual miracles of craniofacial surgery being performed by our special team at the Institute for Reconstructive Facial Surgery at New York University. Headed by Dr. Joseph McCarthy, these surgeons have made some miraculous transformations — both physical and psychological — in children who have been virtual social outcasts because they were born with some distortion or malformation of the head or face. Such surgery is highly complicated and requires teams that could include orthodontists, radiologists, plastic surgeons, ophthalmologists, neurosurgeons, psychologists, anesthesiologists, and others. There are very few centers in the world where such complicated procedures can be undertaken.

Increasingly, these evolving techniques are providing the plastic surgeon with ways of improving the results of jaw surgery performed for cosmetic reasons. Today, the skull and facial bones are being shifted, resized and resculpted routinely and many jaw deformities are being surgically corrected.

THE WITCH'S CHIN

As every child can tell you, the wicked witch in *The Wizard of Oz* can be easily identified by her long, pointed chin.

A condition known as "witch's chin" results when the soft tissue of the chin pad hangs in a lower position than the bony tip of the chin. Typically in such cases, the chin is quite pointed and the point hangs almost straight down. The exact cause of this varies person to person, but the tendency to develop it comes in midlife. It is often a hereditary trait and can be accentuated by the inevitable absorption or shrinking of the jawbone that occurs with age. This happens frequently in people who have lost a significant number of teeth and creates an appearance that is particularly aging. The legendary link of this deformity with the look of witches can be quite distressing.

Fortunately, the witch's chin can be surgically corrected. The technique, from the surgeon's point of view, is not simple, although the operation is of a relatively minor nature as far as the patient is concerned.

The objective of the surgery is to create a forward projection of the chin, thus preventing it from drooping downward, and to fill in the crease on the chin's undersurface. A chin implant is often used, too, along with a rearrangement of the soft tissues. I don't know of more grateful patients than those who, following a successful facelift, find that they still have a witch's chin and undergo a second corrective procedure to eliminate that condition. One such enthusiastic patient told me, "It's like a miracle! It's given me a whole new lease on life."

A Few Words about the Jaw and Orthodontics

Malocclusion of the teeth — either overbite or its opposite in the case of someone with an extreme protruding jaw — is sometimes due more to the malformation of one or both jaws and less to the formation of the teeth themselves, although most people with this condition don't seem to know this. Nowadays, thousands upon thousands of youngsters, and an increasing number of adults, undergo prolonged and expensive orthodontia treatment, enduring months or years of uncomfortable braces, in the misguided belief that this treatment will correct a jaw problem as well as a malposition of the teeth.

Orthodontia is a highly developed specialty which, under the right conditions, can perform wonders. However, while the orthodontist can move teeth, he cannot move the upper or lower jawbones — the maxilla and the mandible. Thus, if the primary aesthetic problem is due to a poorly shaped or positioned jaw, the orthodontia, in terms of that part of the face, will be a waste of time and money. Only direct surgery of the jaws themselves can correct the basic problem and, with it, the external imperfection. In too many cases, the orthodontic treatment brings the teeth into superb alignment while the external aesthetic problem remains.

If you are considering orthodontia for yourself or a youngster in your family, and if you believe the problem of teeth formation is complicated by a receded chin or a protruding jaw, it would be sensible for you to consult a qualified plastic surgeon as well as an orthodontist and consider all the information and opinions before you make a decision about braces on the teeth.

Let's Debunk This Myth

Many years ago there was a cartoon character drawn with an extremely recessed chin. His name was Andy Gump, and he was depicted as a henpecked husband. Even today, common medical parlance describes such a chin as an "Andy Gump deformity." Recessed chins are also referred to as "weak" chins. This is a misconception if ever there was one. I have known people with recessive chins who have been aggressive, persistent, domineering, and strong in both character and performance. I'm sure you have known such people, too. There is not a trace of evidence to support the view that the shape of a person's chin is tied to his or her personality or character.

And much as a receding chin has been, over the years, tied to weakness, pushing one's chin forward has been seen as a gesture of defiance and forcefulness. This, too, has absolutely no link to reality.

However, these myths indicate that the shape and projection of one's jaw do not go unnoticed, particularly if it is too big or too small. So, cosmetic correction for too much or too little is something for people to think about if they have either of these problems.

> "There is one thing that all we women know
> Although we never heard of it at school,
> That we must labour to be beautiful."
>
> — WILLIAM BUTLER YEATS, "Adam's Curse"

Eyelid Surgery | 7

I WAS APPROACHING MY FIFTIETH *birthday, but I don't think that's what brought me to the surgeon's office. Actually, I had been so concerned about the pouches that had developed under my eyes over the last couple of years that I had mentioned them to my internist when I had my last annual checkup. He had explained why this happens to some people and talked about heredity being a factor. I recalled that my father had the same thing and looked like an old man when he was about my present age. It was my internist who suggested — having determined that I was not a big drinker — that plastic surgery might eliminate the bags. He also told me to give up smoking, for lots of reasons (I had heard them all before), including that he felt smoking contributed to the problem. I'm proud of the fact that I did succeed in giving up cigarettes after several unsuccessful tries.*

The precipitating factor had to do with my job. I'm an Executive V.P. with a large conglomerate and I have a good reputation. I've been written up in Fortune *magazine and have had good press notices in the trade journals. The corporation was going to spin off one of their smaller operations into a separate company, and I wanted to head it up. I wanted it so badly I asked the CEO of the conglomerate for the assignment. He didn't know me well, although we had met once or twice, but he did know my reputation and the results of my performance, and though he interviewed me at great length, and I later learned that he considered me seriously for the post, someone else got it. Word got back to me that a rumor persisted in the company network that I was a heavy drinker. Nothing could be further from the truth. I was never a drinker; beyond a drink or two before dinner on weekends, I don't even like liquor. I can't recall that I ever drank at lunchtime during the week, although I always order a drink when others do so at a business luncheon. It usually sits on the table, barely touched.*

Once I got it in my head that this rumor could only be based on my appearance — that is, the bags under my eyes — I was determined to get rid of them, and my wife agreed I should do it. I can't tell you what a difference it's made in my outlook and in my feeling about myself. I wish I could say the happy ending includes my getting the presidency of some other spin-off company, but I can't. However, I know my career is wide open, that I will not be passed over in favor of someone else just because of my appearance. Maybe I'm kidding myself, but when I look in the mirror, I think I look ten years younger. It's been a real shot in the arm and I wish I had done it sooner.

Eyelid surgery is the most frequently performed of all facial cosmetic operations. It is estimated that close to 100,000 of these procedures are performed annually, approximately 14 percent of them on men.

Except for reconstruction of the nose, this type of cosmetic surgery is the most difficult one for surgeons to do, calling for the greatest skill, precision, and judgment. Fortunately, it is also one of the oldest operations in the arsenal of cosmetic surgery and the technique is widely known and practiced.

Early in the nineteenth century, a Berlin surgeon named Albrecht von Graefe introduced a reconstructive procedure designed to help patients who suffered malignancies on the eyelids, which had necessitated the removal of part or all of the eyelid. He called his new procedure *blepharoplasty*, *blepharon* meaning "eyelid" in Greek. Today, blepharoplasty usually refers to *cosmetic* eyelid surgery not necessarily related to a malignancy or other growth that has to be removed.

What this operation does is remove loose and redundant fat, as well as skin, and sometimes even muscle, from the upper and lower eyelids. The effect is often stunning. After full recovery, the person will look rested, clear-eyed, vigorous, and more youthful. Most physicians agree that this operation can do more to make a person appear fresher and younger than any other type of cosmetic surgery. The rest of the good news is that the results of blepharoplasty usually last longer than do those of a facelift or browlift. Removal of eyelid bags is virtually permanent.

Your eyes, after all, are the most expressive part of your body. They tell the world a lot about you. They can be inviting, express fear or anger, give the impression of energy or illness, interest or boredom, intelligence or the lack of it. What makes the eyes so expressive is not the pupil, which merely reacts to light by contracting or dilating, but the movement and appearance of the eyebrows, lashes, and skin around the eyes. We speak of "crinkling" eyes, "laughing" eyes, "doleful" eyes, "cold" eyes, "soulful" eyes, or "calf's" eyes. People often characterize others by their eyes alone. And your eyes are also the first thing that people notice when they meet you, creating an impression that is often a lasting one.

One of my recent patients was a high-powered deal maker with a major movie production company on the West Coast. She was known for her unflagging energy, and she told me that her colleagues jokingly called her "Wonder Woman." Yet, when she came to see me, she said that several people with whom she worked had recently asked her if she had been ill.

This forty-four-year-old woman had never been ill a day in her life — but she could see, when she looked in the mirror, why these friends had expressed concern. The normal effects of aging, coupled with a bout of sleeplessness she had been experiencing, had caught up with her. She told me that she had always had "heavy" eyelids, but that men had often referred to them as "bedroom eyes" and she thought they made her look sexy. But now the eyelids had begun to "bag," giving her a tired look that distressed her. While she had a good marriage, and her husband considered her to be still very attractive, as did her two teenage children, she felt that she couldn't afford to project a tired image in her line of business, where such a premium is put on youth and energy.

I evaluated her as being a stable woman whose expectations about eyelid surgery were quite realistic. She merely wanted to get rid of the bags, and I felt that a blepharoplasty procedure could accomplish this. I booked her for the surgery, the operation went smoothly, and she was well pleased with the results. "I probably could have waited a couple of years," she remarked to me when she came for a checkup several months later, "but I'm glad I didn't. Why live with something so unattractive if you don't have to? Now, every time I look in the mirror I'm relieved to see that those bags are gone."

Let's look at what happens to the body as we age, what makes so many people seek eyelid surgery.

What Age Does to the Eyelids

A layer of fat is normally found inside the bony orbit that surrounds the globe of the eye. It is called *periorbital* fat and is a very important and necessary buffer layer, acting as a shock absorber for the eye inside its bony cage.

As we get older, this fat accumulation tends to increase without any relationship whatever to our body fat. Too much fat, bulging through the skin (which gets thinner and less elastic with age), or merely too much skin or muscle, or a combination of all these anatomical problems, causes bulges in the upper or lower eyelids, or in both. Most people refer to these bulges as "bags," as in: "I woke up this morning with the most awful *bags* under my eyes!" Such bags, also referred to as "pouches" (the technical name is *palpebral bags*) are quite normal — they don't necessarily indicate that there's anything medically wrong with people sporting them. These people tend to be over forty, the approximate age at which this bulging is likely to begin.

Baggy eyelids, especially those that are the result of excess fat surrounding the eyeball, are frequently familial: that is, an inherited family trait. If the characteristic is inherited, it can occur anytime from the early teens onward. In some families, puffy or baggy eyelids can be seen even in quite young children. It is not uncommon for us to operate on patients who are in their twenties or thirties — waiting until middle age in order to get rid of a tired, dissipated look is certainly not necessary.

Sometimes there is an accumulation of water in the tissue, a condition known as *edema,* and when this happens, the eyelid bags are accentuated. In women, edema is usually related to hormonal changes. It is also common in people who drink excessive amounts of alcohol ("gin bags"), who smoke heavily, who have a sleep disturbance, or who constantly burn the candle at both ends and develop a look of chronic dissipation. While the fluid collects throughout the eyelid tissues, it is stored mostly in the fat. Edema fluid will stretch the tissues and this, too, contributes to the formation of baggy eyelids. While fluid collection cannot be corrected by a surgical procedure, reducing the fatty tissue will decrease the potential reservoir for such fluid, thereby reducing the size of the eyelid bags proportionately.

I mentioned "fat," "skin," and "muscle." The muscle involved is called the *orbicularis oculis* muscle; its function is to help close the lids and thereby protect the eyes. This circular muscle squeezes the eyelids closed in much the same fashion as a string would pull closed an old-fashioned coin purse. As we age, this muscle loses some of its tonicity.

In addition to fat, loose and wrinkled skin of the eyelids is also inevitable with advancing age and is greatly accelerated by excessive exposure to the sun and wind. We see it first as small "smiling" wrinkles that appear at the sides of the eyes. Usually referred to as "crow's-feet" (the technical name is *rhytides*), they can be highly distressing when they occur in very young women. Unfortunately, they are impossible to eradicate.

When a marked bagginess of the eyelids develops at an early age — in the twenties or thirties, sometimes even in the teens — it is, as I said before, usually due to a genetic factor. Fortunately, when baggy eyelids occur early in life, the skin and muscle tissue are not yet involved; thus the condition is curable by the simple removal of excess fat.

Katharine Hepburn once said, "Old age is a bummer." Most aging people would agree that it certainly does have its drawbacks. Even gravity is against us. As we age, our eyebrows tend to drop with the pull of gravity. In a small number of patients, lifting of the eyebrows can, therefore, become a necessary part of the eyelid operation, although sometimes it is part of a facelift. In Chapter 10 I'll tell you all about eyebrow and forehead lifts. Suffice to say at this point that this procedure is considerably more extensive than a simple blepharoplasty. However, should your surgeon suggest the procedure as an alternative to eyelid surgery, or in conjunction with it, don't be upset. It's a procedure that's being performed with increasing frequency, and the technique is improving continuously.

In addition to "bags" or "pouches," many people speak of

the "dark circles" under their eyes. This "darkness" is caused by increased pigmentation of the eyelid skin and is usually hereditary. It is more common among people of Mediterranean descent. A common misconception is that blepharoplasty will eliminate such dark skin of the lower lids. Alas! The pigmented skin cannot be totally removed and the circles cannot be wholly obliterated. However, if blepharoplasty is performed for other reasons — to remove bags or pouches — removal of some of the excess skin during surgery can sometimes make the pigmentation less conspicuous, and the overall condition will be improved to a degree.

Candidates for Eyelid Surgery

I have performed eyelid surgery successfully on men and women, Caucasian, black, and Oriental, their ages ranging from the teens to over seventy. Age, sex, and race are not the important factors in determining if one can benefit from blepharoplasty. The important factor is whether the problem can be corrected or improved with surgery.

Although the number of men seeking eyelid surgery continues to increase dramatically, this is still predominantly a woman's operation. While women have, for decades, turned to cosmetic surgery to improve or maintain their looks and their youthfulness, it has only been in recent years that men in any great numbers have felt free to seek this type of help to camouflage the aging process. Women are coming in for eye surgery at an earlier age — many in their early forties, even their thirties. The vast majority of patients range from forty-five to seventy, with a sprinkling of people below, and even above, that age.

Where men are concerned, the eyelid operation has become the most common procedure of all cosmetic surgeries. Many men who still feel shy or uncomfortable about undergoing a full facelift will readily come for a consultation about the possibility of correcting tired-looking, baggy eyelids. Often, such problems are seen by men as having an adverse effect on their careers, or even their love life. After surgery for such problems, men are usually well satisfied with the results and speak of their "increased self-esteem" or having recaptured their "youthful self-image."

Contrary to what some people might think, most blepharoplasty patients are not rich, pampered women with nothing else to occupy their minds. For the most part, they are people who have been active in business or the professions, or in their communities, and probably socially as well. Many are women returning to the job market after having raised a family. They want to continue to look like what they are: youthful, vigorous, often dynamic personalities at the height of their careers and in the prime of their lives; people whose chronological age is out of sync with the age they are able to project. They are most often optimistic about the future.

Ordinarily, eyelid surgery is one of the first cosmetic operations people consider having done, usually before they consider a facelift. It can, however, be done in conjunction with a facelift; it can also be done along with an eyebrow lift. The best candidates for eyelid plasty are men and women with a positive outlook about their future and what surgery might do for them, who are realistic in what they expect from the operation, whose concern with their eyes is not a displacement for some other unhappiness, who have no medical problem that would contraindicate the surgery. If you are thinking of having eyelid surgery, perhaps the most important question you will want to ask the surgeon is this: "Will surgery remove these bags from under my eyes? If so, to what extent?" Then match his answer to your expectations for such an operation and you'll know whether your objectives are realistic.

What Eyelid Surgery Will Do . . . What It Will Not Do

Throughout this book I speak often of patients' realistic expectations about a surgical procedure. Because they undergo surgery to correct some defect or put a hold on the aging process, people should not expect to look like they did in their twenties, or like a movie star, or a prettier sister or friend. Aesthetic surgery can, in most instances, slow down the clock, camouflage the ravages of time, tighten or "clean up" some parts of the face, neck, or eyelids, but it cannot remake you. On the other hand, people who undergo successful cosmetic surgery often find that their personalities and attitudes towards life are, indeed, "remade" — their dispositions improve, along with their self-confidence.

It is important to understand that blepharoplasty cannot eradicate the crinkle lines, or crow's-feet, at the sides of your eyes, nor the horizontal lines that show up when laughing or speaking excitedly. Nor can it fill in or wipe out bags of skin over the cheekbones. While many wrinkles will be eliminated during this operation, many will not be.

Some health problems preclude eyelid surgery. Thyroid disease, both in conditions of hypothyroidism (low thyroid activity) or hyperthyroidism (increased thyroid activity), also called Graves' disease, or thyrotoxicosis, can affect the eyelids. In hypothyroidism, the eyelids become waterlogged and create large bags or swelling of the eyelids that cannot be corrected by surgery. Hyperthyroidism is characterized by both swelling of the lids and bulging of one or both eyes. This condition, too, is not helped by blepharoplasty. The small blood vessels in the retina are affected by any problem of the vascular system, so hypertension and cardiovascular disease can also affect the vessels of the eye, as can diabetes. All of these medical problems are contraindications for eyelid surgery.

Surgeons differ on whether or not they will operate on patients with other eye problems. Many do not recommend surgery if there is preexisting blindness of one eye. I, personally, feel that blindness should not necessarily preclude cosmetic eyelid surgery; however, the risks must be weighed against the benefits. I have operated on people with active and inactive glaucoma, detached retinas, and other eye conditions but, when I did so, it was because the condition was stabilized and the patient's ophthalmologist had agreed to the surgery.

Eyelid surgery is sometimes inadvisable for people who don't produce tears readily. Since the cornea of the eye has no blood supply and is very sensitive to drying, it depends upon the tears for lubrication. Should tear drainage or tear production be diminished even further during surgery, damage to the cornea can result in the form of minute ulcerations. In severe cases, this can lead to scarring of the cornea.

It's essential that you discuss your entire medical history with the surgeon you consult about an eyelid procedure. The vast majority of people who consider this operation are good candidates for it. Here's what happens before, during, and after a blepharoplasty operation.

BEFORE THE SURGERY

Photographs

At the time that you're booked for surgery, you will be scheduled for preoperative photographs to be taken by your surgeon or a medical photographer. The purpose of these pictures is to give your doctor a detailed view of the eyelid area so that he can see what and how much tissue he needs to remove. These photos will go to the operating room with him; they are for *him* — not for your photo album. If you get to see them, I guarantee you'll dislike what you see; but they are essential, much as a chest X ray is essential to a thoracic surgeon. Most surgeons who do not take these pictures themselves will give their patients the name of a medical photographer with whom they are accustomed to working.

Tear production test

After booking you for eyelid surgery, many doctors will have their nurse perform a simple test (known as Schirmer's test) to determine if you have a normal tear production capacity. I said above that failure to produce tears is sometimes a contraindication for this sort of surgery. The test is simple: a very small piece of special paper is inserted onto the lower eyelid to stimulate tear production. Only rarely do we find someone with "dry eyes," and it is my practice to send such people to an ophthalmologist for confirming tests. In many instances, eyelid surgery can still be performed even if tear production is low; but, in such cases, I usually do only the upper or lower eyelids in a first procedure, with the balance of the surgery being performed some weeks or months later.

Medication

Not every doctor prescribes the same medication, but I ask all patients scheduled for surgery to take 1,000 mg. of Vitamin C each day for at least two weeks prior to surgery. This helps in the healing process. To improve clotting, I also prescribe three tablets of Vitamin K to be taken for three days prior to surgery, with the last pill taken the day before the operation. This medication should not be taken by people with varicose veins or a history of phlebitis or coronary disease.

Perhaps the most important of all preoperative instructions about medication is this: avoid aspirin or any aspirin-containing compounds for two weeks prior to surgery and for two weeks after. Aspirin slows down blood coagulation because it interferes with the ability of the blood platelets to agglutinate (or "clump" together), which is the basis of clotting. When the clotting mechanism is interfered with, excessive bleeding can occur during the surgery and can also interfere with healing, creating hematomas (small collections of blood under the skin).

Drugs that contain aspirin or aspirin derivatives include Alka-Seltzer, Anacin, Bufferin, Coricidin, Darvon Compound, Dristan, Excedrin, Fiorinal, Midol, and Percodan. Before taking any medication in the weeks before your operation, read every label carefully or call your surgeon's office if in doubt. Anacin-3 or Tylenol is permissible, should you have need for it. If you take any of the ibuprofen medications, it is probably a good idea to discontinue them for forty-eight hours before surgery, unless they are badly needed for arthritis or other pain.

Just remember: even a single dose of aspirin can adversely affect your blood-coagulating ability.

Smoking

For two weeks before and for two or three days after surgery, you should not smoke. As with aspirin, smoking has long been suspected as a major cause of poor healing. A study of over two thousand patients showed that cigarette smoking was the major cause of serious wound-healing complications in a significant number of cases. Excess scarring is more frequent in smokers than in nonsmokers. Since your cosmetic surgery is for the purpose of improving your looks and overall feeling of well-being, it doesn't make sense for you to fight the very goals that are taking you into an operating room — by lighting up a cigarette during this period.

Where the operation is performed

Blepharoplasty can be performed either in a hospital or on an ambulatory (outpatient) basis. "Same day" surgery is increasing in popularity (see Chapter 4) because of the big financial savings when a patient is not kept overnight. Most ambulatory facilities are well staffed and fully equipped to provide maximum comfort, safety, and satisfaction. Such facilities may be part of your local hospital, separate freestanding clinics built especially for this purpose, or even part of a doctor's well-equipped office.

Hospital stay If the surgery is performed in a hospital, you can be discharged in 24 to 48 hours. The principal reason for remaining in the hospital is so that you can be kept under observation for complications that are possible, although unlikely to occur.

If the operation is performed in an ambulatory facility, you will be kept in a recovery room for one to four hours, until the effects of the anesthetic wear off.

About the Anesthesia

Anesthesia for eyelid surgery can be either local or general, depending on your preference. A common misconception is that you need to be partially awake to help the surgeon by moving your eyes. Such is not the case. However, a deep anesthesia, the kind administered in abdominal or heart surgery, is not necessary, either. When a general is used, it's usually a light anesthesia, augmented by a local anesthetic that contains Adrenalin, which helps stem bleeding from the small blood vessels. Whichever you choose, the anesthesia will probably be an intravenous drug, along with oxygen. Gas inhalation is rarely used.

If your surgeon expresses a strong preference for one type of anesthesia over the other, I'd be inclined to go along with his choice. However, if you, too, have a strong preference that differs from the surgeon's, the final decision should be yours. Both forms of anesthesia are safe and equally satisfactory for a blepharoplasty.

One factor you may want to consider is that a general requires the services of an anesthesiologist, who assumes responsibility for managing your whole body health during the procedure, including the administration of oxygen if necessary. The services of an anesthesiologist are not included in your surgeon's fee — you pay according to the anesthesia fees that are the going rates in your area. If you opt for the local, it is usually administered by the surgeon and there is no additional fee for that part of the procedure. Rest assured that a local works well and that you will be relaxed and comfortable throughout the operation. In many cases, little or nothing of what went on in the operating room is remembered by the patient.

So, listen to your doctor's opinion; ask as many questions as you like; then make your choice.

Paying Your Bills

In most instances, medical insurance will not cover cosmetic blepharoplasty unless the bags hang down over the lash margins so that they actually interfere with vision. Most insurance companies require medical proof that such interference with the eyesight is the true reason for seeking a surgical procedure. Such proof usually consists of a thorough ophthalmologic examination. Photographs can also be used as suitable evidence, but they must be standard medical pictures and they must show at least 3mm coverage of the upper part of the pupil by the sagging upper lid. *Ptosis* (or sagging) of the upper eyelids, and *ectropion*, the loss of tone that causes sagging of the lower eyelids, are also covered by most medical policies, but these ailments must also be documented. A patient's statement that vision is obstructed is not deemed sufficient evidence for the insurance carrier.

As with most cosmetic surgery, you will probably be asked to pay the surgeon's fee in advance of the operation. If you have an anesthesiologist, his bill will be sent to you shortly after the surgery — possibly given to you while you're still in the hospital or the ambulatory facility. If your medical policy doesn't cover the hospital charges, it is quite likely that you will be asked to bring a certified check to the hospital upon admission.

The Blepharoplasty Technique

The usual purpose of the blepharoplasty operation is to remove redundant fat and loose tissue from the upper and/or lower eyelids. If both the upper and lower eyelids are involved, the operation will last between one and two hours, with the lower eyelids taking most of the time. From a technical point of view, the lower eyelids are usually more difficult to correct.

When you arrive in the operating room you will be tranquilized and sleepy, but not totally asleep. Possibly you will be aware of your surgeon drawing lines on your upper and/or lower lids. He is simply measuring and marking the exact location of the incisions and the amount of tissue he plans to remove.

At this point, if you are under local anesthesia, your surgeon may give you a little more drug, intravenously, to relax you further, although he will not put you to sleep completely. Drugs such as Valium are used for this purpose. Given intravenously, these drugs often produce amnesia, so it's quite possible that you will have no recollection of the rest of the procedure.

Under local anesthesia you will probably feel a small needle prick on each side of your face, near the eyelids, followed by a slight burning sensation, which is mildly uncomfortable. This is merely the local anesthetic being injected. Should you elect to have a general anesthetic, you will feel the anesthesiologist make an intravenous injection in your arm, and that's all you'll remember until you wake up in the recovery room.

Where the Incisions Are Made

A simple incision is then made in the upper lid, placed so that the scar will be in a natural fold and well camouflaged after recovery. If only a moderate amount of excess skin is slated to go, and if it's in the middle of the eyelid, the incision will be shorter — perhaps no more than two to three centimeters in length — approximately an inch. In young people there is usually very little skin to remove. But if the excess skin extends to the corner of the eye — usually the case after middle age sets in — then the incision is longer, extending out and into the crow's-feet. Often there is a considerable excess of muscle and this is removed along with the skin. After the skin has been cut away, the excess fat that has amassed beneath it is also removed.

The incision in the lower lid also varies in length, depending on how much tissue must be cut away. The surgeon places this incision along the first natural line just below the lower eyelashes, usually about 1 to 3 mm — approximately a tenth of an inch — below, and continues it to the edge of the lid closest to the nose, finishing the incision by extending it to the crow's-feet, or into a natural laugh line.

After the lower incision is made, the skin and muscle are gently separated and "teased" away from the fat that lies underneath. This fat is then removed. It is this part of the procedure that calls for considerable skill by the surgeon, because taking away too much fat can cause a patient to have "sunken" eyes.

The excess skin and muscle are then pulled up carefully and removed — cut away. The lower eyelid incision is then stitched together. After full recovery, it is usually very difficult to detect where the incisions were made.

Now let's examine what happens after the operation.

AFTER THE SURGERY

Bandages — Bandaging the eyes is not necessary, although some surgeons prefer to apply a slight pressure bandage for a few hours to minimize swelling. Whether or not a bandage is applied, your eyes will be lubricated with a comforting ointment after surgery.

Pain — There is rarely any pain after a blepharoplasty. However, as you would expect, there is some mild discomfort and a feeling of tightness. Neither is very distressing and both will be short-lived.

You may experience some irritation of your eyelids, manifested in itching or by a burning sensation, perhaps even some redness of the whites of the eyes. These symptoms are usually related to the fact that patients are unable to close their eyes completely during the period immediately following surgery. As a result, the air dries the cornea and a dry cornea is certain to induce irritation. (This is a reflex action that nature has created to help obtain more tears, which serve to wet the cornea and protect it from drying and injury.)

To prevent such symptoms, or to treat them if they occur, I usually prescribe a bland, artificial tear ointment such as *Lacrilube* or *Durilube* (your doctor may suggest other good ones) to be squeezed into the eye each night until all symptoms have calmed down, or until the eyes can close completely during sleep. It is also a good idea to use artificial teardrops during the day. Only two or three drops about four times a day are necessary. There are several excellent artificial tear products on the market and your doctor can recommend one, if needed. Two that I recommend are *Hypotears* and *Preferin Liquifilm*.

Bruising

A certain amount of swelling and discoloration (or "bruising") of the eyelids can be expected. The swelling usually subsides after a few days; the bruising normally disappears within two weeks. However, bruising is unpredictable; it varies, person to person. In some people it can last longer than two weeks. Most likely, however, you can be back at work in as little as three or four days, wearing sunglasses or even tinted glasses to hide the bruises and discoloration.

Wearing sunglasses

I advise my patients to wear sunglasses — the wraparound Porsche-type glasses are excellent for this purpose — for seven to ten days, both to hide the effects of the surgery and to protect the eyes from sun, dust and other irritants. After ten days, lightly tinted glasses suffice. However, when the swelling is at its maximum, you should avoid wearing dark glasses over long periods of time since the pressure of the glasses can create swelling on the upper cheeks.

Makeup

If you prefer to wait until you can use makeup comfortably before returning to work, allow ten days to three weeks. By that time, wearing makeup, it will be hard for anyone to detect that surgery has been performed. Do not apply makeup if all the small crusts have not fallen off the scars. Some people find the crusts are gone in as few as ten days — others find it takes a bit longer. But when they're gone, you can use mascara, eye shadow, lash liner — the works!

Makeup should be removed with oil pads or light cold cream. A light moisturizer may be applied, but avoid heavy creams, especially overnight.

Appearing in public The eyes of most blepharoplasty patients look quite presentable in ten days. A small number of patients find they need more time than this because their healing process is slower. This is due to no fault of the surgeon or the patient — it's just that each person's rate of healing is different and unpredictable.

Ice compresses After you leave the hospital or ambulatory facility, ice compresses may be applied to your eyes for a few minutes at a time, several times daily, to reduce any discomfort or swelling. After twenty-four hours, the compresses can be discontinued, since they will no longer be effective.

The ten days after surgery On the second or third day, most people can watch television and even do some reading.

For ten days after surgery, it is a good idea to sleep with your head elevated on one or two pillows, and on your back, if possible. However, turning from side to side is permissible. It's also quite important to avoid a head-down position for long periods of time, as the force of gravity will tend to increase the swelling. A good rule of thumb is to keep your head above the level of your heart. When bending, bend at the knees.

You may cleanse your eyes with cotton and warm water one week after the surgery. Avoid washing the eyelids with soap and water for two weeks after the operation, as your eyes may not be closing fully and the soap will irritate them.

Since alcohol tends to increase fluid accumulation in the tissues and, therefore, promotes swelling, avoid all types of alcoholic beverages for a full week after the operation.

No strenuous activities are permitted for three weeks following surgery. This includes intense exercise, jogging, swimming, sports, dancing, and "working out." Sex, which is more strenuous than you might think, is not a good idea for the first week.

Getting your hair done

One week after surgery, you can shampoo your hair in the shower, keeping your head back, not leaning forward. Your hair can be blown dry, with the temperature setting on the blower turned to "Warm." If possible, get someone to blow it for you to avoid a lot of movement of the head and even of your arms.

Removal of stitches

Stitches are removed three to five days after surgery. Some surgeons like to replace the stitches with a temporary paper-tape strapping in order to give the wounds continued support. The tape, when used, is removed in a few days.

Sunbathing

It's OK to sunbathe one month after surgery, but avoid getting sunburned. Use a good sunscreen on the scars. I recommend a total block cream or, at minimum, a No. 15 sunscreen.

Contact lenses — Contact lenses can be inserted as soon as the incisions are healed and the lids can be stretched sufficiently to permit manipulation. This occurs approximately two weeks after surgery. However, a certain amount of tightness of the lids is to be expected for several weeks, or even months, after the operation. Most patients who wear contact lenses feel comfortable with them within the first months. If you feel any discomfort, postpone wearing them for another week or so, or until there is no longer any discomfort.

Postoperative depression — As the aftermath of most cosmetic surgery, many people suffer a period of slight depression while they are recuperating. Fortunately, this is only temporary and will disappear as unexpectedly as it came. Don't worry over this mild feeling of letdown. It's understandable. After all, you went into the operating room as a healthy person, wanting to look better. Now, when you look in the mirror, instead of a happy transformation, you see scars, discoloration, maybe some swelling. Take heart — this part of the recovery period will pass quickly, and soon you will see the remarkable and pleasing results of your eyelid surgery.

THE SCARS

During the first three to five weeks after your operation, the scars may become red and a bit lumpy. This is a normal process as the scars "mature." These symptoms will go away.

It takes several months for the scars to fade and it is not uncommon for some to remain red for six months to a year. Usually, eyelid scars behave extremely well and end up as fine, white lines. It is important to remember that scars are always permanent, no matter how carefully the incisions are stitched. For practical considerations, however, they present no problem. For one thing, the eyelid skin enjoys a unique ability to heal with less scarring than almost any other skin area of the body. Second, your surgeon will place the incisions in the natural folds of the skin so that they won't be conspicuous.

Women, of course, enjoy the added advantage of being able to use makeup. Men who undergo blepharoplasty end up with the same scars as women, yet even without makeup, the scars are barely visible.

The Possibility of Complications

Some patients are acutely aware of even minor and temporary problems; others tend to be more stoical and hardly notice them. For example, some people experience a slight decrease in visual acuity for a while after the operation and worry about it; others with the same symptom assume this to be a logical postoperative symptom. This minor disturbance usually goes away within hours; perhaps it can take a day. It's related to swelling and, often, to the protective ointment that's put in the eye at the end of the procedure.

A high percentage of patients are unable to shut their eyes completely during sleep for the first few weeks after surgery. This condition is quite normal — nothing to be alarmed about. In a small number of patients (perhaps 2 percent to 5 percent) this persists for months. In very rare instances, it remains a permanent condition.

Complications that could threaten vision are extremely rare. Visual problems that do occur happen during the first twenty-four hours after surgery.

While blepharoplasty doesn't change the shape of the eyeball, it does temporarily change the way the lid fits over the eyeball. In the early phases of the healing process, some thickening of the scar tissue in the incisions takes place and, at that time, they pull like rubber bands that are being stretched. With the passage of time and softening of the scars, the rubber band effect diminishes.

In some patients, a type of distortion that makes them look a bit unnatural, somewhat starry-eyed or wide-eyed, results from what we call "scar pull." Just as soon as the scars soften and the body absorbs them, the natural expression returns. This complication does not happen very often, and when it does occur, the scar pull will disappear in three to four months. Slightly tinted glasses are an excellent means of camouflaging such a temporary condition.

One complication after blepharoplasty that is more serious is a marked pulldown of the lower lids so that the white of the eye (the *sclera*) shows. This can be the result of excessive swelling (*edema*) in the tissues, in which case the condition will be temporary and subside in a few days, although it could last a few weeks. If, however, the surgeon removed too much skin or muscle, or both, during the operation, this condition (ectropion) could be permanent. When too much tissue has been cut away, repair of the sagging lid can be extremely difficult and the results obtained are not always perfect. Skin grafting and other reconstructive procedures may be required. Your best protection against this complication is to select a surgeon who has had a good deal of experience performing blepharoplasty. This is not a procedure that should be performed "on occasion" by any surgeon. It requires proper training, a finely honed skill, and the experience that comes of continuing performance of the operation.

Occasionally, small cysts develop in the suture areas. These are harmless and can be removed easily as an office procedure. Infection in the eyelid area is very rare, although it can occur if a patient rubs the eyelid with a dirty hand.

Permanent blindness following blepharoplasty is extremely rare. It's been reported in only a few patients out of many, many thousands of people who have had the operation.

Any surgeon's practice will yield a very small percentage of patients in whom unsightly scars develop. When there are such scars, a minor, secondary corrective procedure is required to trim them away. This is usually done on an ambulatory basis, and most surgeons do not ask for an additional fee to perform the second surgery. Though secondary corrective procedures might *improve* bad scars, nothing eliminates scars completely.

Debunking a Few Myths

There are some misconceptions that keep some good candidates for eyelid surgery from having the operation.

One such myth is that once you have surgery on your eyelids, you have to have it done again every few years. This is untrue. A good eyelid plasty should last for many years — as many as ten to fifteen years in some people; or virtually the rest of one's life.

Another myth is that eyelid surgery will change a person's vision. While it's true that if you wear contact lenses you'll have to give them up for a few days or weeks after surgery, (or until the lids have healed sufficiently for you to get the lenses in and out without discomfort), it is untrue that your eyesight will be affected by a blepharoplasty.

Another rumor is based on half-truth: you can never go in the sun again after an eyelid operation. For about a month after surgery, it's a good idea to stay out of the sun, as the wounds are too new to tolerate the sun's rays. But after that, it's perfectly OK to sunbathe, using a sunscreen on the scars, or wearing dark glasses.

One of the most intriguing myths is that eyelid surgery can slant your eyes — give you eyes like Sophia Loren's. I wish I were able to do that, but I can't. Nor can anyone else. While the surgery often does make your eyes appear larger, it doesn't change the basic shape of your eyes.

However, the *opposite* of the "Doctor, make me Oriental eyes . . ." myth happens to be possible. Blepharoplasty is performed frequently in the Orient to create a Western-type crease or fold in the upper lid. It is the pull of the *levator* muscle attached to the skin that creates the crease or fold in the upper eyelids of Caucasians. In most Orientals, this muscle is not attached to the skin. To create a Western look, the edges of the muscle are actually attached to the skin with stitches.

Looking to the Future

It is never possible to predict the exact duration of results from any cosmetic procedure, but we do know that the results of blepharoplasty are long-lasting. Ten or even fifteen years is a

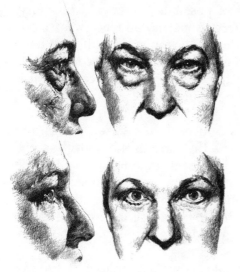

In late middle age, this patient developed marked eyelid bags, complicated by some skin wrinkling. The result shown was achieved by a blepharoplasty.

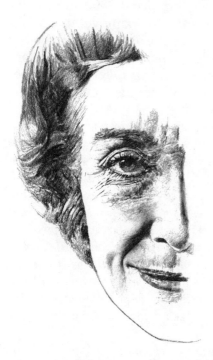 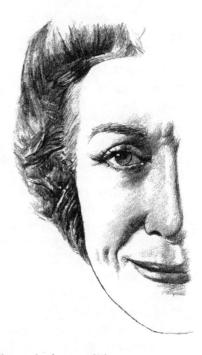

The entire facial expression can be brightened after eyelid surgery.

time span that's in the realm of possibility — even probability. Of course, people age at different speeds, and no two friends should expect to experience the same results, even if they have the same surgeon and are the same age. For someone whose problem is simply bulging of the eyelids due to excess fat, it is likely that the results will be permanent.

Eyelid surgery gives you a good deal more than just a pretty, or handsome, face. Having a noticeable decrease in bags and wrinkles around the eyes means the sand in the hourglass will appear to move more slowly for years to come. Every look in the mirror provides reassurance that you have regained some of your fresh, youthful appearance. To someone who dislikes the signs of aging that can be noticeable around the eyes, this can serve as a great shot in the arm, in terms of optimism about the future.

Patients, young and old alike, who have had this type of facial surgery say they *"feel* more alert because (they) *look* more alert" and they describe their after-surgery personalities as being "rejuvenated," "rekindled," and "revitalized." I had a sixty-year-old woman patient recently, a hardworking volunteer at a suburban hospital. Recently widowed, she expressed the feeling that she would never again be the woman she *had* been before her husband passed away, but that she was determined to become a "new" woman and get on with her life.

I had large pouches under my eyes; I had great bags <u>above</u> my eyes — one great big bag above my right eye and two bags above my left eye. I had wanted eye surgery for years . . . certainly a minimum of five years. After my husband passed away, I realized there were a lot of things in my life that needed to change. Changing the way my eyes looked was one of them. All I was hoping was that I would not look quite so old around the eyes and not have those circles and pouches. I didn't want to look sweet sixteen; I just wanted to look a little better.

I had gotten so I would not look at myself in the mirror. If I looked in the mirror, I would look at my hair, or look at my lips if I were putting on lipstick, but I would not really look at <u>all</u> of my face. I tried to ignore the actuality. I realized I had been doing that for years. I just couldn't stand the way I looked.

<u>Now</u>, I guess I can't really remember the way I <u>did</u> look. I've seen some pictures of myself from before, and there's a world of improvement.

What I had hoped for was to renew my passport for the rest of my trip through life. I think I accomplished that. It gave me a new lease on life.

Another blepharoplasty patient, a thirty-nine-year-old paralegal aide who worked for a large metropolitan law firm and was taking graduate courses at night in the hope of some day entering law school, had this to say about her surgery:

My mother had droopy eyelids, and I could see even when I was a teenager that mine were going to be the same. It really bothered me. When I was in college, a lot of the kids were using eye makeup, but it didn't make me look good — it just accentuated my problem. I don't think there was ever a time in my life when I didn't wish that this problem would disappear.

This year, as I approached my fortieth birthday, I got anxious about growing old, and since any unhappiness with my appearance had always centered around my eyes, I finally decided to see a doctor. Once the ball was put in motion, it kept rolling along and I had a mixture of apprehension and excitement that I would finally unload those droopy eyelids.

The operation was easier than I thought it would be. I had it done as an outpatient, with a local anesthetic, because I didn't want to think of it as such a big deal. I had arranged to take my annual three weeks vacation after the surgery, and I spent most of it at home, wondering if I had done the right thing because, frankly, in the first two weeks at least, you don't look so hot. A few times I went to a department store and wandered through the cosmetic section. I bought almost fifty dollars' worth of eye makeup as a present for myself, to use when the eyelids were healed.

Almost everyone noticed a change in me when I went back to work, but not a single person seemed to realize what it was due to. I was very surprised. Everyone attributed the change to the new makeup and to my having had a long vacation. Once all the bruising was faded, I started to feel really terrific. I found myself looking in the mirror a lot, and I liked what I saw. I had never disliked my other features, and now I think I'm kind of nice looking. I'm well satisfied with myself. I think it's made me more outgoing with people because I'm no longer self-conscious about my looks. I only wonder why I waited so long to do it.

"If the nose of Cleopatra had been shorter, the whole face of the earth would have been changed."

— BLAISE PASCAL, *Pensées*

"He that has a great nose thinks everybody is speaking of it."

— THOMAS FULLER, *Gnomologia*

Rhinoplasty: Reshaping the Nose | 8

*I*T'S CHANGED MY LIFE. *As simple as that. I hated the nose I was born with from the very first day I looked in the mirror and recognized that my nose had a decided hump on the bridge. No one else in my immediate family had such an ugly nose. But my grandfather had it, although, being a man, I don't think he cared that much about his looks. His generation didn't pay that much attention to what they looked like. My generation is different. Even the boys care about their hair and their skin and their clothes and even their noses. I know two boys my age who have had their noses fixed.*

Anyway, I hated it. From the time I was about twelve or thirteen I knew that I was going to get my nose changed. I didn't have to bug my parents. They agreed I should do it. It was a sixteenth-birthday present and I wouldn't trade it for a convertible.

The operation wasn't bad, and anyway, that's not what's important. What's important is that I now have a nose I can live with. If you want to know the truth, I'm actually pretty. *You can see for yourself. If you could see my old pictures, you wouldn't believe it's the same person. From ugly to pretty. That's me.*

I met Lady Bird Johnson at a party in her honor in New York in 1984. The hostess introduced me as a plastic surgeon. After chatting a while, Mrs. Johnson asked me if I would have accepted

115

her as a patient for nasal plastic surgery when she was much younger. "Could the bump have been taken out?" she asked me. "Yes," I told her, "no problem."

"I always hated this nose," she said. "When I was young, I didn't know anything could be done about it and I'm not sure I would have had the courage to do it if I had. But certainly, had I known that I would one day be the First Lady, there is no doubt in my mind that I would have had it changed."

Mrs. Johnson's comment that when she was young she didn't know anything could be done about the nose she disliked is a comment typically made by people of her generation. Today, however, with cosmetic surgery a much-discussed topic on television talk shows, in magazines, and in news reports about celebrities who have undergone nose operations, just about everyone is aware that an unattractive nose can often be improved, sometimes remarkably so, through plastic surgery. More than half of all cosmetic procedures on the face are nowadays performed on this feature. Since the beginning of this decade, the number of such operations performed annually has tripled, with over 100,000 of them now done each year, one-fourth of them on men.

The nose is the most prominent feature of the human face, and, though the eyes reveal a great deal about a person's emotions and inner feelings, it's the nose that is the feature most likely to be mentioned first if one is called upon to describe someone's looks. A writer or commentator describing an actress or other public personality might speak of her nose as "Grecian," "tilted," "impertinent," "innocent," "crinkled," "pug," "retroussé," "Etruscan," or "sensitive"; a man's nose might be described as "protruding," "hooked," "pendulous," "sniffing," "lavender-tinted," "aquiline," "eaglelike," "bulbous," "handsome," or "classic."

The list of adjectives describing the nose goes on and on because our genes, which determine the look of the nose, are most inventive when it comes to designing this feature. Like our fingerprints, no two are exactly the same. They differ in size, in the thickness and shape of the bones and cartilage, and in the skin texture. Even if two noses were similar in appearance, they would look different because they'd be surrounded by different eyes, brows, chins, ears, and a difference in the overall contour of the face and skin color.

Unfortunately, nature is not always compassionate when handing out noses. Truly unattractive noses, some more easy to alter than others, can be found on otherwise pretty girls and handsome men.

Corrective surgery of the nose to improve functioning or to reshape its appearance is known as *rhinoplasty*, *rhin* being a form of the Greek word for "nose." There is historical evidence that plastic surgery was done on the nose for cosmetic purposes as much as 2,500 years ago. Modern rhinoplasty goes back about a hundred years, with techniques modifying and improving all the time. Our society goes through phases in terms of what it considers beautiful in a nose. There are nose fashions much as there are fashions in clothing or hairstyle, though not to the same degree nor with the same rapidity of change.

Rhinoplasty was first introduced in the United States in a serious way in the thirties. The early results were often characterized by removal of too much, resulting in many retroussé (turned up) noses — also referred to as "scooped out," "ski jump," or "Bob Hope" noses. Many were overshortened. Many had a "pinched" look. In some, the nostrils were elevated too much. Such noses grew to be the vogue in the thirties and forties, a style imposed by the surgical procedures themselves. Since, in many cases, the operation succeeded in removing a large hump or hook, patients embraced the procedures wholeheartedly and were willing to settle for what they got — often, an artificial-looking nose. The current trend is to correct less, rather than more, so that the results are pleasing and subtle. Today, reconstructed noses tend to look softer, more like they belong where they're found and less like they've been transplanted.

CANDIDATES FOR RHINOPLASTY

The human nose changes in shape until a person reaches physical maturity. Until recent years, there was a generally held belief that nose surgery should be delayed until the age of sixteen or seventeen for girls and a year or so later for boys. We now believe the nose is fully developed in most girls by the age of fifteen or sixteen, sometimes even by fourteen, and in most boys by sixteen or seventeen. However, through the years, the aging process continues to affect the nose, as it does all other facial features.

In due course, it may become longer when the skin loses some of its elasticity, or gravity may cause the tip to evince a drooping tendency.

Rhinoplasty in adults — even some over forty — can have excellent results and can bring such joy to so many people that we'd be foolish to deny them this opportunity for improving their looks, self-assurance, and overall sense of well-being. The important thing is for the doctor and would-be patient to explore thoroughly the reasons why the surgery is desired, why it was delayed so long, what the likelihood is for a good psychological adjustment to the new nose, and how willing the patient is to accept the surgical risks that increase with an older person.

I well remember Mary-Kay, an army nurse who had seen service during the Korean war and who came to me in the late fifties after deciding to return to civilian life. Despite the fact that she was a fairly large woman, her nose dominated her face to such an extent that one barely noticed her beautiful green eyes and her high cheekbones and good jawline. She told me she felt she was embarking on a new chapter in her life, that she was going into an administrative job in a Dallas hospital and was very excited about her second career. Mary-Kay had always disliked her nose, hated it, in fact, and said she had joined the army because she thought of herself as ugly and felt her so-called ugliness would, in civilian life, stand in the way of her being successful, either in her career or in her social life. I recall her saying, "I thought I could get lost in the mass of the army and that a uniform could stop people from looking at my face."

Mary-Kay had made many good friends in service and her excellent record and promotions gave her a sense of achievement and self-confidence. She had never married and felt that a better nose would make her prettier and help her embark on her new career with confidence in her appearance. I thought her an ideal candidate for rhinoplasty. She was very positive about what she hoped to achieve through surgery. "I'm past the age where I'm going to win any beauty contests," she told me; "I just want to see a nice face when I look in the mirror." She also had the sunniest of dispositions: she laughed easily, was quick with a clever retort when the occasion permitted, and went into surgery absolutely certain that she would be content with the results. And she was!

I didn't create a small nose for her; she didn't have the face for it. But by eliminating the sizable hump and creating a fine, straight-line nose that fit her face and size, she did become a strikingly attractive woman. Shortly after I discharged her as a patient, I received a note from her. "I am happy," she wrote, "happier than I've ever been. I'm still 'me'; but now I like the looks of 'me.' "

The Right Candidates for Rhinoplasty

Like Mary-Kay, the best candidates for a nose operation are people who are physically well, psychologically stable, realistically expectant about the results of such surgery, and, of course, people who have anatomical problems that can be helped by rhinoplasty.

Although the so-called best age for a cosmetic nasal operation is in the late teens, no age precludes this type of elective surgery if all other physical and psychological factors favor it. However, older people have to consider that bones grow more brittle as we age and that, during surgery, there is a possibility that the bones in the nose might break in several places rather than along the exact fracture line planned for the procedure. Should this happen, it's not a disaster, but it certainly makes the procedure more complicated. Also, the skin of the nose has less elasticity, so, if a major reconstruction of the underlying skeleton is undertaken in an older patient, we can't count on the skin to shrink to the form of the new skeleton as promptly as it does in most young people. Sometimes, in older patients, we find it necessary to make some external incisions and remove some skin. This is no big deal except that it does leave a visible scar over the top of the bridge of the nose.

These relatively minor drawbacks notwithstanding, the main factor in deciding whether to have rhinoplasty if you are middle-aged or older, is whether you are likely to have the capacity to adjust to your new changed appearance. A noticeable facial change in a fully matured individual is more likely to draw comments from relatives and friends than it would with someone younger. If you fall into the "mature" category and are contemplating rhinoplasty, you should know that such comments are sometimes negative ones, and you should be prepared to take them in stride. You should also ask yourself if you are prepared to abandon your old self-image since you've lived with it so long. Teenagers and people in their twenties usually have no problem with this.

Today, there are more men seeking to have their noses reshaped, and they make excellent candidates for this operation. They usually state that they just want to look "better" or "maybe a bit more handsome." I have never had a male patient who sought the "perfect nose."

What People Want from Rhinoplasty

Among men and women seeking this type of cosmetic surgery, the most common request is for a reduction of part or all of the nose. This may simply involve the removal of a strong hump. When a nose with such a hump also has an enlarged tip, the nose appears to "hook over" when the face is animated. Another popular request is for some improvement in the size and/or shape of the tip of the nose. In many patients, the *only* desire is for a reshaping of the tip.

The lowermost dividing portion that runs from the tip of the nose to the upper lip and separates the right nostril from the left is known as the *columella*. This structure, too, is frequently a cause of unhappiness, particularly if it hangs down. Other complaints include protruding or plunging nasal tips, excessive size or flaring of the nostrils, and too much width along the base of the nose where it joins the cheeks on either side. There are also numerous deformities of the septum, the partition inside the nose that divides it into two cavities and can affect its appearance.

Requests to build up noses that seem too small to their owners are much more rare than requests to reduce the nose size. Noses can, indeed, be too short, too flat, or the bridge may be depressed in what is known as a "saddle" nose. Such noses can be reconstructed using grafts or implants. In a graft, a small piece of bone or cartilage is taken from another part of the body and transplanted to the nose. An implant involves placing an inert plastic substance, such as silicone, under the skin. Both techniques have their advocates, with implants favored in the

Orient. However, the overwhelming majority of plastic surgeons prefer cartilage or bone — living tissue — for such implants.

Anatomy of the Nose

The nose is an organ with several distinct functions. Foremost, it is a complex air-conditioning apparatus and an airway to the lungs. It filters and cleans the air we breathe. It humidifies and preheats it. The sense of smell is also an important function of this organ, although it is far less developed than in animals. Finally, the nose has a major influence on vocalization and phonation. A change in the nasal passages will alter the tone and timbre of the human voice.

Rhinoplasty is the most difficult of all cosmetic facial operations. Not only is it technically challenging, but it is not always possible to accurately predict the results. The surgeon must first conceptualize the operation in terms of the small and compartmentalized structure of the nose. Then, since it takes a minimum of a year for the tissues to heal totally and for all traces of swelling to disappear, the surgeon must visualize not only the immediate, but also the long-range results — what the nose will look like and how it will fit the face a year or more after the surgery. This is a complex challenge.

It is helpful to compare the structure of the nose to that of a tent, the shape of which is mostly determined by the framework which supports it. How the fabric stretches to become a tent depends, in large part, upon the tent poles, which can come in many sizes, shapes, and thicknesses. The thickness and resiliency of the fabric are also important factors in determining how the tent will look. Like a tent, the nose has an underlying framework — the bone and cartilage which we call the skeleton of the nose. (It is medically known as the osseocartilaginous structure — *osseo* for "bone"). The skin is stretched over the top of this framework.

Much of what happens in a rhinoplasty operation is determined by the shape of these "tent poles" and by the thickness, resiliency, and elasticity of the skin that covers them. During the surgery, the skin covering is lifted off, just as a tent fabric might be. The tent poles and crossbeams (bone and cartilage) are then reshaped, sized, and literally sculpted to assume the desired shape. The fabric, or skin, is redraped over the new framework.

Imagine a tent that is covered by a very thick tarpaulin impregnated with oil and difficult to bend or work with. When placed back on the new framework, it fits poorly over the new shape. Or, imagine the opposite: a skin that is pliable, thin, and easily draped over the poles.

This analogy gives you some idea of what a surgeon anticipates he will need to work with when he examines a potential candidate for rhinoplasty. In six out of ten people whom I interview for this surgery, the results are quite predictable, and I can clearly visualize the noses I will be able to shape. The other four are people whose results are less predictable because they have anatomical conditions that limit the degree to which I can achieve optimal results. This is not to say that such people should forgo rhinoplasty; on the contrary, we can often make a person quite happy with the results that *are* obtainable. An important part of the surgeon's job during a consultation is to help patients understand what objectives are realistic for them.

Many people who come for a consultation with a preconceived notion of the type of nose they'd like to have are surprised to learn how many factors determine whether the nose of their choice is possible: the shape of the bones and cartilage, the shape of the face, heredity, age, and — probably the single most limiting factor — the skin, if it is thick, coarse, and oily. No matter what the shape of the bone and cartilage structure, it may be difficult, if not impossible, to drape thick skin over a reshaped cartilage. Every nose has a certain unique combination of all these anatomical characteristics which influence the outcome of surgery. However, no one should disqualify herself, or himself, as a good candidate for rhinoplasty without consulting a plastic surgeon. What may appear to you like a nose unsuitable for reconstruction may appear to a surgeon as quite suitable indeed.

Something that often surprises patients is learning from the surgeon that an alteration of the size and shape of a nose should be accompanied by appropriate changes in other facial structures, such as the jaw or chin, if the best results are to be obtained. We often augment or alter the chin along with the nose, particularly if it is recessed or small in size. Your surgeon's evaluation of your entire facial structure will determine whether a secondary procedure is advisable.

Understanding the Limitations of Rhinoplasty

The greatest surgeon in the world, whoever and wherever he is, cannot create a beautiful nose out of anatomy that does not have suitable potential for it to begin with. A nose is not a piece of clay or a block of wood that can be sculpted to suit the wishes of either patient or surgeon. For the surgeon, rhinoplasty is the most humbling of all aesthetic operations because, since it is performed internally, through two nostrils, it is like decorating a room to which the only access is a mail slot in the door. Rhinoplasty is a "feel" operation — the surgeon must learn to feel what he is doing, often without clearly seeing what he's working on.

As I explained earlier, certain types of skin make it difficult to achieve the results we might wish for. Another anatomical feature that precludes optimum results is a "short" columella. Seen in profile, the columella projects slightly below the nostril rims where it curves gently. Some people have what we call a "hidden" columella; when the face is viewed in profile, it is hidden behind and above the nostrils so that they appear to be hanging downwards like a curtain. In recent years, we have developed techniques for correcting this condition, but patients who have it should not expect rhinoplasty to give them the nose of their dreams.

Contraindications for Rhinoplasty

More difficult, sometimes even impossible to correct, is the nose that not only has a short columella but which is also notably foreshortened so that its tip appears to be "tethered" — it does not project forward in a natural way. What the surgeon must attempt to do in such cases is to try in every way possible to create a natural-looking projection of the tip. I regret to say that, despite every technical advance known to surgery at this time, the result of such operations is severely limited, at best.

The patient who has a combination of thick skin and a short

columella presents the surgeon with an anatomical situation that is virtually impossible to improve. In most such cases, an experienced surgeon will advise against surgery.

A frequent cause of nasal obstruction, and by far the most common cause in adolescents, is *vasomotor rhinitis*. This is the medical term for stuffy nose due to swollen membranes. The symptoms are not caused by bone or cartilage obstructing the passageways. The condition is usually intermittent and travels from side to side, often seasonally or related to emotional stress. It is particularly common in teenage girls, this being the time in life when hormonal influences are at their maximum. In such cases, the ailment is usually self-limiting and clears up when the teen years are over. Vasomotor rhinitis is not curable by surgery and can even be aggravated by it, at least temporarily. Hay fever and the common cold are other frequent disorders that cause nasal obstruction. Rhinoplasty is usually postponed during the acute phase of a cold, or until these temporary symptoms disappear.

Often, it is extremely difficult for someone who has wanted nasal reconstruction for a long time to understand why a surgeon, or several, advises against it. Almost nothing invokes my compassion more than a teenage girl who, after months of anticipation, has finally arrived at my office to make arrangements to correct a nose she truly dislikes, only to be told that she will have to live with it for the rest of her life. How difficult it is to explain to her that the results of surgery could well make her more unhappy with her looks than she is now!

Consoling a patient for whom rhinoplasty can do nothing is one matter. Dealing with that person's family is another. I have, on more than one occasion, incurred the wrath of parents who are unable to accept my advice to forget about surgery. They simply cannot comprehend why plastic surgery, which can perform miracles for people with deformities due to burns, birth defects, accidents, and so forth, cannot improve an unattractive nose.

If the first surgeon you consult advises against rhinoplasty, by all means get a second opinion. If, however, the second surgeon concurs with the first, I suggest you accept what you've been told and concentrate on making the most of your other features — lovely hair or beautiful eyes, or a good figure.

The daughter of hardworking middle-class parents from Brooklyn, Laura was not a very attractive girl. Her face was round and pudgy, full of sixteen-year-old baby fat. Her nose was bulbous and her skin was coarse and oily. She also suffered from severe acne. Laura was so emotionally charged, so full of anticipation when I saw her, that I dreaded having to tell her that the results of nasal surgery would not be satisfactory at that time, due to the combination of problems affecting her skin. To compound the problem, she had two friends who had benefited greatly from rhinoplasty, and I had operated on *both* of them. "Neither of my friends' noses were as ugly as mine," she pleaded, "so you should be able to do more for me than you did for them." It seemed to her that the uglier the nose, the more improvement should be possible. If Laura was incredulous, her mother was downright hostile. "Tell me," she said, "do you only operate on people who already have beautiful noses?"

I wanted to leave Laura with some hope; I simply couldn't send her away from that consultation as distraught as she was. I suggested she should wait a bit, that as she matured, both her face and her skin would change and perhaps I might be able to improve her nose in a couple of years. This was true: as teenagers shed their baby fat and the face takes on the lines of a matured person, and as acne improves or disappears, it is sometimes possible to make additional facial improvements with rhinoplasty. I suggested she come back in a year or two so that we could reevaluate her situation. I never thought she'd take me up on it.

Four years after that traumatic consultation, Laura returned to my office, this time without her mother. She was now twenty and had a good job as a researcher with one of the major publishing houses. I didn't recognize her. She was smartly dressed, with the mandarin collar of her soft blouse framing a thinned-down face. She had let her rich, black hair grow to shoulder length, and she had apparently learned how to use makeup to good advantage. Her acne had disappeared with the baby fat. She looked like an entirely different person, although she still had a nose too large for her face.

"Doctor," she said, "I waited longer than you suggested and here I am. I have gotten myself together and I have a good job. I have a wonderful boyfriend who teases me sometimes about my nose but he does it lovingly so I don't mind. I have to say I'm pretty happy, but if you can make any improvement at all in my nose, I'd still like to ask you to do it. I'll be satisfied with even a small change for the better."

I operated on Laura and there was a definite improvement. She was very happy with the results. She has married her "wonderful boyfriend" and has advanced to group supervisor in her company. As I write this, she is expecting her first child in five months. "If she has my old nose," said Laura in a letter to me, "I want you to promise to put her on your list — no matter how long you make her wait for the operation."

Assuming you or someone close to you is a *good* candidate for nose surgery, let's examine what lies ahead in terms of preoperative preparation, the procedure itself, and postoperative care and expectations.

BEFORE THE SURGERY

Photographs — When your doctor books you for surgery, you will also be scheduled for preoperative photographs to be taken by a medical photographer or by the doctor himself. These highly detailed photographs are essential to the surgeon's total evaluation of your facial structure and helps him plan certain technical variations in the procedure. Like chest X rays for a thoracic surgeon, the photographs are an important part of the operation. They are not meant to flatter you, and if you get to see them, I'm certain you won't ask for copies for framing. Postoperative photographs will also be taken, but not for many months, perhaps as long as a year after the surgery.

Medication — I prescribe for my patients 1,000 mg. of Vitamin C each day for at least two weeks before the operation. This helps in the healing process. I also prescribe three tablets of Vitamin K to be taken for three days prior to surgery, although this medication should not be taken by anyone with varicose veins, a history of phlebitis, or coronary disease.

The most important piece of advice I can give you about taking medication is to avoid aspirin or any aspirin-containing drugs for two weeks prior to, and for two weeks after surgery. Aspirin slows down blood coagulation because it interferes with the ability of the blood platelets to clot. When clotting is interfered with, excessive bleeding can occur during surgery and can hinder the healing process.

Aspirin-containing drugs or compounds that you should avoid during this period include Alka-Seltzer, Anacin, Bufferin, Coricidin, Darvon Compound, Dristan, Excedrin, Fiorinal, Midol, and Percodan. Anacin-3 or Tylenol may be taken. Bear in mind that even a single dose of aspirin can create a problem. If you are on prescription drugs, be sure to check with the prescribing doctor or with your cosmetic surgeon on whether such drugs contain aspirin or aspirin derivatives. If you take any of the ibuprofen medications, it is probably a good idea to discontinue them for forty-eight hours before surgery, unless they are badly needed for arthritis or other pain.

There are other drugs in popular usage today among joggers and other athletes, as well as among people who suffer from arthritis. These, too, should be discontinued for two weeks prior to surgery because they also inhibit coagulation. Among these are Clinoril, Feldene, Naprosyn, and Indocin.

Smoking

Because smoke acts as an irritant to the nasal passages and could create a lot of discomfort and even some unnecessary bleeding, you will be advised not to smoke for a minimum of two weeks *after* surgery. Like aspirin, smoking is suspected as a major cause of poor healing. (See p. 49 for information on a study of cigarette smoking and its effects on scarring, healing, and complications after surgery.) Therefore, as you approach the date for your rhinoplasty, ask yourself if that isn't as good a time as any to give up smoking permanently. If you give it up, the day will come when you'll look back on the operation as the time when you became *healthier* as well as better looking.

Allergies

It is, of course, optimal if hay fever sufferers can have their surgery during a quiescent period. However, from a practical point of view, such timing is not always possible because surgery, in young people at least, must often be done during school holidays, such as spring and summer vacations. Fortunately, with modern drugs (particularly steroids), we are able to operate on allergy sufferers, and they go through the procedure and postoperative period quite comfortably. Even severe asthmatics need not forgo rhinoplastic surgery. We usually postpone an operation during the first one or two days of an acute respiratory infection, especially if the patient is running a temperature. Several days' postponement, until the acute phase of the cold has passed, is optimal.

Where the operation is performed

A rhinoplasty can be done either in a hospital or an ambulatory facility, which would have special operating rooms that are, nowadays, frequently a part of a doctor's offices. Sometimes, such facilities are attached to a hospital, or they are freestanding clinics set up for this purpose.

Should you go into a hospital, the length of your stay there will be one to three days, which includes the day prior to surgery, when you're admitted for routine tests. As an outpatient, you'll be kept in a recovery room for approximately four hours after surgery and then permitted to go home.

There is a current trend towards having cosmetic surgery done on a "same day" ambulatory basis because hospitals have become so expensive and patients usually have to pay for their stay out of their own pockets. However, some people do feel more secure in a hospital setting and others with complicated nasal problems or with general health problems may feel better in a hospital.

ABOUT THE ANESTHESIA

The rhinoplasty procedure can be performed under local or general anesthesia. Because of its simplicity, most surgeons prefer to use local anesthesia combined with preoperative sedation and additional sedation, if necessary, during the course of the operation. Under a local anesthesia, you will not be fully awake. You will be calm and very sleepy but aware of sounds, manipulation, and the general goings-on in the operating room. But you will experience it all in a haze or fog, and there will be little or no memory of the operation.

A general anesthesia may be suitable for people who are very nervous about the idea of surgery and who might be comforted by the knowledge that they will be "asleep" for the entire procedure. When a general anesthesia is used, it's usually a light one, augmented by a local anesthesia that contains Adrenalin, which helps stem bleeding.

While the final choice is up to you, you should consider your surgeon's reasons if he prefers one type of anesthesia over the other. If he has a strong preference, it's usually a good idea to agree to his choice, unless your own strong preference runs counter to his.

One of the factors you'll want to consider is that a general anesthesia requires the services of an anesthesiologist, while a local is usually administered by the surgeon. The anesthesiologist assumes responsibility for managing your whole body health during the procedure, and his services are paid for in a fee that is separate from that of your surgeon. Since cosmetic surgery is rarely covered by insurance, this second fee may enter into your choice of general vs. local. Either type is safe and comfortable.

Paying Your Bills

Although most cosmetic surgery is not customarily covered by medical insurance, rhinoplasty is one of the gray areas between pure reconstructive surgery and cosmetic surgery. A patient with an unattractive nose suffers every bit as much as a patient with any other facial deformity, whether it is congenital or caused by injury.

Almost everyone seeking a nose operation has been coached by a friend or relative to say they have breathing trouble. "I have a deviated septum, doctor," is the usual opening remark in a first consultation on rhinoplasty. It is well known that most insurance companies will provide some coverage for the so-called deviated septum — *provided* it truly obstructs breathing.

The truth is that about 75 percent of us have deviated septums — it is the norm, not the exception. The septum, made of bone and cartilage and covered with mucous membranes, is the partition that runs down the center of the inside of the nose and divides it into right and left chambers. A deviation means that the septum is bent or deflected to one side. If a deviation is severe, it can cause blockage of one or both nasal airways and, as the natural air flow is hampered, a true health problem can result.

In actuality, the deviation that is present in most noses rarely reaches a degree at which breathing is affected. I assure you that the insurance companies know this, as do all plastic surgeons. When preparing a patient's medical history, a physician can usually determine whether there is a significant nasal obstruction or whether breathing difficulties, when they exist, stem from allergies or other ailments.

Many people believe that an injury or fracture in childhood can be the cause of a nasal hump in adolescence and that it should be compensable by insurance. Ninety-nine times out of a hundred the insurance companies will say no to this. First, a bump on the nose that is scheduled to show up in adolescence will show up at that time whether the teen had a childhood injury or not. In no way has it been caused by falling out of a sleigh or crib.

There are some rare and unusual situations in which a severe childhood injury — perhaps one suffered in an automobile accident — can cause deformity of the nose. But such problems are usually troublesome and obvious prior to adolescence.

Should you want your surgeon to support your contention that the nose operation is necessitated by some childhood injury, he will have to provide suitable documentation to the insurance carrier. The insurance companies investigate each case, and the burden of proof is on the documentation you and your surgeon provide. Should your particular situation turn out to be compensable, it will be one of the rare instances when this occurs.

As with all cosmetic procedures, the surgeon's fee is payable in advance of the operation. If you have an anesthesiologist, his bill will probably be given to you before you leave the hospital or ambulatory facility, or mailed to you shortly thereafter. If you go into a hospital for your operation, be prepared to have the hospital ask you for a certified check upon admission.

The Technique

The only preoperative preparation will be for you to wash your face thoroughly with soap and water, using pHisoHex or some other antibacterial soap. This is to be done about twelve hours before surgery and again immediately before it. Some physicians prescribe a preventive (prophylactic) antibiotic, particularly if there are infected acne pustules on the face.

The operational technique varies from person to person, depending on what the patient and the doctor would like to achieve and on the anatomical characteristics of the person's nose and skin. There are, however, some basics that apply to all rhinoplasty operations. The procedure is carried out inside the nose; except in rare instances, no external incision into the nose is made. Almost always, the technique calls for the surgeon to separate the skin from the underlying bone or cartilage and mucous membrane.

A bony and cartilage protuberance on the nasal bridge (a "hump") is removed with either a chisel or a rasp. If the nose is too broad, the nasal bones are surgically fractured and then molded into the slender shape that is desired. Either before or after this remodeling of the skeletal structure of the nose, it is usual to reduce or reshape the cartilages that form the tip of the nose. The exact order of these steps varies according to the problem in the individual patient and, of course, according to the technique of the surgeon. Nothing is more pleasing than a natural-looking nasal tip, but remodeling the tip of the nose is the most technically difficult part of the procedure. Tip revision requires precise separation of the cartilage from the overlying skin, followed by very exact sculpting of these two paired, wing-shaped structures into a new and more pleasing shape. Sometimes it is also necessary to add small pieces of cartilage that were removed while reducing the nose, or the surgeon must reduce the septum to improve small imperfections in the tip of the bridge.

If the nostrils appear too flared or rounded, or are too big in proportion to the new nose size, a "piece of pie" may be removed from the base of the nostril to reduce and reshape this structure. This procedure does result in a small scar at the base of each nostril, and they are permanent but rarely noticeable. In any event, it is a necessary trade-off, and I have performed it in approximately 14 percent of my rhinoplasty operations. Some surgeons actually perform such alar base resection (the *ala* is the edge of the nostril) in over 90 percent of their rhinoplasties.

Finally, the incisions are stitched together with very fine sutures. Most surgeons use an absorbable suture material, such as catgut, inside the nose and it dissolves and falls out by itself, saving the patient the minor unpleasantness of having it clipped out. However, when it is necessary to perform a small external incision in each nostril, these sutures must be of the non-absorbable type, usually nylon, and have to be removed in three or four days. But don't worry — even this removal is not painful.

You'll recall that I compared the nasal skin and the underlying skeleton bone and cartilage to a tent with its tent poles. When the skin over the bridge of the nose is thin, it easily covers the new underlying framework. But, closer to the tip of the nose, the skin becomes thicker and sometimes adjusts poorly to the sculpted cartilage beneath. The result is a distinct lack of shape, often a pudgy look, with a tip that is too round.

The duration of the surgery depends on the scope of the operation. It usually takes from half an hour to an hour and a half.

THE SCARS

Since rhinoplasty is performed from inside the nose, there are no postoperative scars — except where the nostrils have been reduced. As I said, such scars, at the base of each nostril, are permanent but virtually unnoticeable.

AFTER THE SURGERY

Bandages

At the end of the surgical procedure, your nose will be lightly packed with gauze, and a splint dressing will be applied on the outside to protect your nose and reduce swelling. The splint will be held in place with tape.

Pressure bandaging of the eyes is advocated by some surgeons, but I believe it is uncomfortable and probably serves no purpose.

The nasal pack, if your doctor used one, will be removed either forty-eight or seventy-two hours later. (A few surgeons do not use packs.) The trend is towards the use of very small packs, except when extensive work has been done on the septum, in which case the packing may remain in place anywhere from three to five days.

The protective splints will be removed in seven to ten days. After that, all dressings, splints, and packs are gone. If "permanent" stitches were used in each nostril, those will be removed before the first week is over.

Pain

Rhinoplasty is not a painful operation. You may be uncomfortable for the first day or so, but pain is minimal and easily controlled by mild painkillers. The local discomfort depends on the amount of packing that's used. If tighter packs were necessitated by extensive work on the septum, the discomfort might be increased. Some people do experience a dull headache and, since the packing makes it necessary to breathe through your mouth, you will have some dryness and irritation of the throat.

Swelling and discoloration

For the first forty-eight hours after surgery, you can expect quite a bit of swelling and black and blue around the eyes. This happens in about half of all patients, and it's not possible to predict who the escapees will be. Most patients look much worse than they feel during the first couple of days.

There are no secrets about how bruising can be prevented. Various drugs such as steroids, enzymes, and antihistamines have been touted as effective, but there's no solid clinical evidence that they are.

Ice compresses applied to the eyes may be helpful in holding down the oozing from the small blood vessels beneath the skin, which is what causes the discoloration. We're not really sure how effective the compresses are, but since they do no harm and make some people feel a bit better, we suggest them. They can be discontinued after forty-eight hours.

The signs of bruising disappear in about ten days, although there are rare instances when they last longer. It will, however, be at least a year until all traces of swelling disappear, and that is approximately when the final results of your surgery will be apparent.

The tip of the nose holds its swelling the longest and is subject to the greatest fluctuations, usually related to changes in the weather, to menstrual cycles, and to episodes of acne, sunburn, or even emotional upsets. All this calls for patience!

If your rhinoplasty is performed during cold weather, it is advisable to have the heated air in your home appropriately humidified to prevent your mucous membranes from drying out.

Bleeding

A certain amount of bleeding from the nostrils is usual for the first twenty-four to forty-eight hours after surgery. For this reason, a "nasal diaper" is put in place to catch the small amounts of blood. This dressing must be changed frequently. The amount of leakage varies from person to person and, to a degree, depends on how much surgery was performed. If there was a good deal of work done on the septum, the bleeding is apt to be more than just the usual annoying trickle.

More vigorous bleeding from one or both nostrils can occur but is uncommon. When it does occur, it is most likely to be during the first forty-eight hours after surgery or during the first week, and again at about the tenth day. We have found that those patients who tend to be hyperactive and don't take it easy during the first week or so are more likely to have a "bleed." Such bleeding is usually of little consequence and stops by itself provided the patient remains quiet and keeps her or his head in an elevated position. Occasionally, if the bleeding is persistent, the surgeon will repack the side that is bleeding with a small cotton pack soaked in Adrenalin, which helps to stem bleeding. It is exceedingly rare that a blood transfusion is required.

Nasal congestion Some temporary obstruction of the nose is very common after a rhinoplasty because of coagulated blood or crusting along the incision lines and because the lining of the inner nose is swollen. There is likely to be some congestion for several weeks, but it will come and go. The sensation is similar to having a very mild cold or hay fever, and when the swelling both inside and outside the nose diminishes, so will the congestion. There have been cases where some congestion persisted for as long as a year or two, but this is exceptional.

Blowing your nose Don't blow your nose for three weeks after your operation. After the splint has been removed, you may clean inside each nostril once a day with cotton-tipped applicators soaked in a solution of one-half hydrogen peroxide and one-half water. This is to be done until you are again permitted to blow your nose.

| *Bed rest and diet* | Except for going to the bathroom, complete bed rest is prescribed for the first two days after surgery. And, to cut down on the possibility of bleeding, your head should be elevated on two pillows.

Since chewing requires some extra facial motion that could promote bleeding, you should consume only very soft foods (soup, soft-boiled eggs, cooked cereal, Jell-O, ice cream) and liquids (except for alcoholic beverages) for the first forty-eight hours. Since your sense of smell and taste will be diminished during this period because of the nose packing, foods will lose their appeal, anyway. Many patients report, often with joy, that they lose a few pounds during this period. Rarely does anyone complain about the curtailed diet.

Washing your face and hair; wearing eyeglasses | Following removal of the splint, wash your nose gently twice daily with soap and water. If you find your nose tends to be very oily, use an astringent after washing to control the oil production. Good skin care is very important at this time. If the pores become blocked with oil, the reduction of the swelling will be much slower.

Your hair may be shampooed on the day the splint is removed. Put your head back, not forward. You'll find shampooing easier in the shower than in a washbasin at the beauty parlor. Dry under moderate heat.

Do not allow eyeglasses to rest directly on your nose for six weeks following surgery. They can rest on the splint, or their weight can be supported with strips of paper tape attached to the skin of the forehead after the splint is removed.

Physical activity

Some surgeons limit the physical activity of rhinoplasty patients quite severely for many weeks or months. I find this unnecessarily restrictive. I tell my patients that three weeks after the splint is off they can swim, jog, golf, play tennis, or ride horseback. Body-contact sports such as volleyball, football, hockey, wrestling, and so on are prohibited for six months.

After six weeks, the nose is as healed as it will ever be. Even the fracture lines are healed by then. This doesn't mean that I'd send you into a boxing ring where someone would be aiming for your nose. A direct blow to the nose could dislocate it, of course.

After the packing and splint are gone, a small amount of sunbathing is permissible. But be certain you don't get sunburned.

Injury to the nose

If your nose suffers some injury after rhinoplasty — certainly something to be avoided if at all possible — treating it so that it resumes its preaccident condition is more easily accomplished than had a similar injury occurred in an accident *before* the operation. The reason for this is that a nose which has been deliberately fractured by a surgeon almost always breaks along the same lines as the surgical fracture. For a surgeon, it is not too difficult to simply push the displaced nose back into position, under anesthesia, of course.

While few people ever suffer such injuries after rhinoplasty, I mention this because the fear of it happening is quite common and if you're contemplating the operation, that unlikely possibility should not deter you.

What you'll see in the mirror

It's important for you to realize that the final results of a nasal operation are not always those visible to you in the mirror after the dressing and splints are removed. If your skin is thin and your bones reasonably delicate, you might look terrific even this soon after surgery. On the other hand, if your skin is on the thickish side, you might look as though a professional boxer had taken a swing at you and connected right to your nose. My point is this: you have to be patient. Most of the swelling and discoloration will disappear — probably all of it, in time — but it will be many months before you see the ultimate result.

In any event, you will look much better when a week or two have gone by. If your nose looks absolutely terrific when the splint is removed, be prepared for it to swell up somewhat and maybe look worse a few days later, since it is the splint that works to hold down the swelling. Once it is removed, the tissues can fill up with water and appear swollen. You may not know what the final shape of your nose will be like until many months later — more likely, a full year later.

I mentioned the swelling and bruising, but in addition to a face of rainbow hues, it is also possible that you might have some skin irritation where the tape held the splints in place. But I assure you that, once you've overcome the shock of that first glimpse in the mirror, you'll see your face change for the better day by day and with it will come a growing satisfaction that the operation is over and done with . . . and that the improvement made it definitely worthwhile.

The Year Following Surgery

Once the packings and splints are gone, you will probably see your surgeon once a week for several weeks. The intervals between checkups will then grow longer, and about a year after surgery, you'll have your final visit with your doctor. The fee for follow-up visits is usually part of the initial fee you paid the surgeon for the surgery.

By the time your first postoperative year has gone by, you will be quite accustomed to the "new you" and, if you're like most rhinoplasty patients, you'll barely remember what your face looked like before your nose was reconstructed. (Several years after rhinoplasty, most people cannot even describe what their nose looked like before the operation.) Many patients say something like this: "My nose blends into my face so well that it seems like it was always that way."

The Possibility of Complications

Fortunately, the great majority of postoperative complications that could follow rhinoplasty are of a minor nature and require no correction, or a minimal, secondary operation to tidy them up.

Occasionally, a hematoma (a small blood clot) will develop inside the nose, but this is not a serious complication. Should this happen, your doctor will determine whether to leave it alone until it's absorbed by the body, or aspirate it when you see him in his office.

Minor changes in the skin, such as small burst capillaries and tiny blemishes, are not uncommon, and sometimes they are permanent. But they are a small price to pay for good results in changing an unattractive nose into an attractive one.

Infection following rhinoplasty is very rare. Sinus infections can flare up, although they rarely are the direct result of the operation. Most often, when they occur, they are due to abnormalities of the internal structure of the nose. Infections are treated with appropriate antibiotics and sinus drainage if called for.

I mentioned earlier that a small amount of bleeding does occur in the first day or so after surgery and that this is normal and of no consequence, even if your surgeon has to repack your nose. Very rarely, however, a nosebleed can be significant and require more medical care, possibly even another trip to the operating room. However, only twice in many thousands of rhinoplasty operations have transfusions been necessary in my practice. The risk of this happening is very small.

The most common of the significant complications is the "overoperated nose." The trend today is away from this towards *under*operating so that the reshaped nose looks like it belongs on the face. In fact, the best outcome of rhinoplasty is not a perfect nose, or even a near-perfect nose. It is an attractive one that fits the face so well it does not suggest that surgery was ever done.

Sometimes rhinoplasty doesn't achieve the best result possible, and one of the most common causes of such failure is the surgeon's desire to get that so-called "perfect" result. Often, this goal is simply impossible to achieve. Both surgeon and patient have to accept the fact that there will be limitations on what can be accomplished. Such acceptance not only prevents subsequent disappointments but also leads to a more natural-looking nose.

Approximately 5 to 10 percent of rhinoplasty patients ask that the newly shaped nose be changed again. Sometimes the surgeon thinks that further improvement can be made in a second procedure, and even the most skilled rhinoplasty surgeons do perform minor secondary corrections in about 5 percent of their patients.

Revisions, however, are more difficult to do than the original surgery; they should be delayed as long as possible following the first operation in order to permit the swelling to subside and the wound scar to mature. Six months is considered a minimum wait by most doctors, but there are no hard rules on this. It varies with the patient and depends on a number of factors, the principal one being how rapidly the person recovers completely from the original operation. Sometimes, during this waiting period, a person will decide she or he likes the new nose after all and doesn't want a revision.

Should there be a small residual lump or bump on the nose, it can usually be scraped away in a second operation, usually a minor procedure. Sometimes a slight unevenness of the tip calls for correction. In rare instances, the bones that were fractured and repositioned during surgery "wander" slightly and an adjustment becomes necessary. In my opinion, a surgeon should not charge for such secondary procedures, provided the patient brings it to his attention within a reasonable period of time.

They made a handsome couple, Mr. and Mrs. Talbot of Locust Valley on the Long Island shore of New York. She was fair, freckled, dressed in country tweeds, and very aristocratic looking. They were both in their thirties: he a lean, sun-bronzed and well-groomed stockbroker, who flew his own plane; she a mother of three children, a golfer and bridge player, active in church affairs.

Her nose was a bit long, with a very high hump on the bridge. "I have always hated my nose," she told me, "ever since I was twelve years old and this bump appeared. That bump comes from my father's side of the family . . . they were from Scotland and they all had it. I wish my father hadn't passed it on to me. I wish I could have inherited my mother's lovely small nose."

I pointed out to her that a high rise on the bridge of the nose is very characteristic of Anglo-Saxons and is considered aristocratic and quite handsome by many people.

"Perhaps," she answered, "but not on women."

I asked her what kind of nose would make her happy, fully expecting her to reply that she wanted a straight, but still long, nose — but one without the bump, a nose to fit her tall, rangy body. "Small," she told me without hesitation. "I want a very small nose."

I described to her what I thought could be accomplished. I suggested she should have a nose a bit smaller — but not by much — than the one she now had; slightly turned at the tip, but by no means pug, with a graceful, almost straight, bridge. I emphasized that, in my opinion, her nose should still be slightly on the long side to fit the angles of her face.

We all seemed to agree, including her pin-striped husband. Mrs. Talbot's operation went smoothly; the postoperative course was uneventful. One week later I removed her dressings and splint. Even at this very early stage the nose was clearly a success. It was almost exactly the nose I thought we had agreed upon.

At this point, most patients are either deliriously happy or puzzled at what they see in the mirror. Rarely is any patient totally without emotion or some expression of satisfaction or dissatisfaction. But the Talbots were silent. Stony. No comment of any kind. In subsequent visits to my office, my nurse and I tried to convey our own pleasure with the result. We never got any comment from the couple. They routinely showed up for her checkup visits, were polite and proper, but there was never a clue as to how either of them felt about the results of the surgery.

Six months after the operation, I received a phone call from Mr. Talbot. He told me that his wife was very unhappy with the outcome of the rhinoplasty but had been hesitant about calling me. I was thunderstruck because I considered that the result of her surgery was among the best I had achieved that year. "Bring her in," I told Mr. Talbot. "Let's see what we can do."

I was amazed when I saw Mrs. Talbot. Her nose was truly beautiful. It was graceful, elegant, slightly long, with a straight bridge on profile. A minimal tilt at the end. I would be happy, indeed, if I could do this well for every patient.

"Please, Dr. Rees," she said, "you must help me. I chose you as a surgeon in the first place because I had heard you try to please your patients. This nose is not what I wanted, not what I asked for. I am simply miserable with it." I looked at her husband. I met an expressionless stare. I had no hint as to whether or not he agreed with his wife. I was unable to convince her that, by any standards, her nose was a triumph of the art of plastic surgery. It fit her face, her figure, her style. It was aristocratic, well shaped, and there was no hint at all that she had been operated on.

"You don't understand," she told me, "My mother was Irish and she had an adorable turned-up nose. That's what I always wanted."

I pointed out, as I had before the surgery, that she had a long face with finely chiseled bones and told her that a small, turned-up nose would be inappropriate. But she emphatically

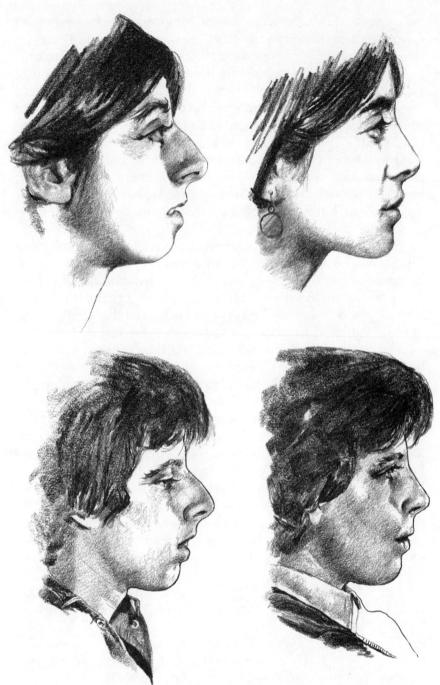

Rhinoplasty will frequently change a teenager's entire facial expression.

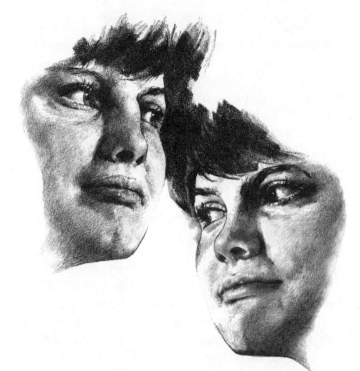

Lowering the bump on the nose is particularly effective for patients with "pert" noses.

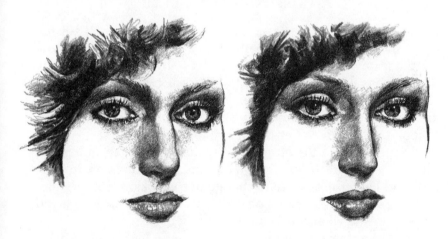

A beautiful woman troubled by a slight bump in her nose underwent rhinoplasty. Her nose was shaved and narrowed slightly. Sometimes a small modification can make a major improvement in a person's looks.

wanted her mother's nose and told me flat out that if I didn't create it for her she would find someone else who would. It was then that her husband commented.

"She'll get what she wants," he said. "You might as well be the one to do it. She does like and respect you."

I did considerable soul-searching and finally, with reluctance, booked her for another operation. I turned up her nose, shortened it more, and created a gentle ski slope. I hated that operation. I almost hated myself for having agreed to do it. My main job, I reasoned, is to make people happy with the way they look. So I turned her into a tall, elegant lady with a small, turned-up nose. She was deliriously happy. Her entire attitude seemed to change. She was full of smiles, bubbly with enthusiasm, warm to my staff when she came for her postoperative visits. She had her hair cut short and took to wearing makeup for the first time.

When we had our final consultation before discharging her as a patient, she reached for my hand and held onto it. "Dr. Rees," she said, "you've given me exactly what I wanted. Now I look like my mother instead of my father. I have a perfect Irish nose."

Twins and Rhinoplasty

During my years of practice, I have had the opportunity several times to operate on one or both of a pair of twins. The attitude of twins towards cosmetic surgery has always fascinated me. Sometimes, twins — particularly identical twins — identify so closely with each other that they want to look alike, dress alike, and remain that way. Both may seek rhinoplasty, but they want to look exactly alike after the operation as well.

In other cases, the struggle of twins to attain an individual identity, separate from that of the sibling, creates an intense desire to have rhinoplasty to change one's looks. On more than one occasion, I've operated on one twin while the other delayed surgery to see what the first outcome would be.

I recall a pair of identical twin girls who had come in with their mother for consultation. They were exceptionally pretty despite the fact that their noses were uncommonly large for their faces, with prominent humps and an unattractive way of plunging downward when they smiled. One of the sisters wanted surgery; the other was strongly opposed to it both for herself and for her twin. During the consultation it became clear that this split opinion had become a major point of friction within the family.

Against her twin's objections, I operated on the sister who wanted the rhinoplasty. The result was very natural looking and turned the girl into a true beauty. The other girl continued to proclaim her resistance to changing the shape of her nose.

Eight years later the second twin asked for a consultation. Both sisters had married; both were mothers. She confessed to me that all these years she had been jealous of her sister's looks after the surgery, but because she had taken such a strong stand against the operation, she had felt obliged to stick to her position. She admitted she had wanted rhinoplasty all this while. I performed pretty much the same operation that her sister had, and I'm delighted to say that the results were equally successful. The second twin was ecstatic, as was her entire family.

Debunking the Myths about Rhinoplasty

If I've heard it once, I've heard it a thousand times: "Doctor, isn't it true that rhinoplasty causes the nose to drop?"

This is a common misconception and a difficult one to put to rest because it is so pervasive. What is true is that our bodies react to the forces of gravity throughout our lives and, just as the face, and women's breasts, sag or seem to fall with age, so does the tip of the nose tend to slide southward as the years go by. The rhinoplasty operation certainly does not accelerate the process; nor does it bring it about in any way. In fact, the small amount of scar tissue that results from the operation will, in most instances, inhibit dropping of the nose.

In the rhinoplasty procedure, the surgeon usually overshortens the nose the slightest bit because, when the tissue swelling subsides, there is a certain amount of "settling" that takes place during the first few weeks. The nose continues to "settle" for many months, but imperceptibly so. This is all part of the postoperative recovery process. Of course, as the rhinoplasty patient grows older, the nose will show a tendency to drop, exactly as it might in a person who did *not* have nasal surgery, although it will be less noticeable in the person who had the operation.

That surgery causes an interference with breathing is another myth. Unless there was a preexisting problem that could, in some way, be exacerbated by the operation, it is very uncommon for any breathing problem to be created by the operation. In fact, some people find that their breathing is improved by it. As I pointed out, nasal stuffiness is common for a few weeks after surgery, but this is more like a cold or hay fever and is due to the swelling of the membranes inside the nose.

In general, however, those with problems of breathing before rhinoplasty — allergies, hay fever, hormonal influences, or emotional stress can all cause such problems — are not going to be cured by this operation. But it won't make them any worse, either. When someone has a truly deviated septum or an unusual bone formation that has made breathing difficult, the operation *can* make some improvement.

Another myth, one that frequently discourages professional singers from undergoing rhinoplasty, is that increased nasality can be induced by the surgery. Changes in resonance, timbre, and nasality of the voice, especially the singing voice, can indeed occur, but negative changes are exceedingly rare. In fact, the reverse sometimes happens: much to the delight of a singer, his or her voice becomes less nasal and more resonant.

In describing your postoperative period, I listed the physical activities you can engage in after rhinoplasty and explained that some surgeons are more restrictive than I am about sports and exercise. I think that such severe restrictions serve to perpetuate another myth: that the nose is exceedingly fragile after cosmetic surgery.

The simple facts about healing do not support this belief. Though it has been fractured, the nose is about as soundly knit at six weeks as it will ever be. The bones of the nose never do knit together as firmly as do the leg or arm bones. They are thin, delicate structures that heal by a layer of scar tissue, which joins together the fractured edges. Every once in a while, the bone bridges this fracture gap and heals over solidly; more often than not, the fracture lines remain forever united by scar tissue. The reformed nose is not made of glass or eggshell. It is no more vulnerable to injury than a nose that has not been operated on.

Another myth tells us that if a rhinoplasty is unsatisfactory, it cannot be repaired. As I discussed earlier, secondary procedures may sometimes be necessary and can often be helpful in creating a nose that is well liked by both patient and surgeon. If you opt for rhinoplasty, let's hope you like the result well enough so that you never need to consider a secondary operation. But you should know that minor corrections *can* be made.

Here's something else you shouldn't believe: "I can always spot a nose job . . . you can't fool me!"

We can, and do, "fool" people much of the time. Successful rhinoplasty produces a nose that looks so natural no one can recognize that surgery has been performed on it.

In the last fifteen years, we have perfected many significant aspects of rhinoplasty technique, not the least of which is the art of underoperating. While in some patients certain anatomical characteristics preclude the creation of a nose that's completely natural looking, the majority of patients emerge with results that are, after full recovery, undetectable to anyone but the most intimate of friends or relatives — and sometimes not even to them if they haven't seen the patient during the postoperative period of swelling and discoloration.

Looking to the Future

When it comes to satisfaction with the results of a cosmetic procedure, nothing ranks higher than the joy and gratitude of young patients who have replaced a hated nose with one that makes them feel better looking and more satisfied with their looks. Later in life, rhinoplasty can be equally rewarding, but it is the young who quickly forget their former self-image and replace it with a new, more comforting one that they will carry with them for the rest of their lives.

Every surgeon who performs successful rhinoplasty operations will tell you about striking personality changes that often occur after this procedure. Many people blossom after a nose operation, so much so that the preoperative personality virtually disappears, to be replaced by a new one that often leads to other changes: in grooming, bearing, disposition, and outlook on life. A new sense of improved self-confidence is the most frequently observed change. I have received many letters from previous patients telling me of the changes they experienced after their successful surgery. Nothing is more gratifying to a doctor than to learn of happiness brought about by a much desired change in looks as the result of a cosmetic procedure.

I am moved to tell you about a recent patient, an extraordinary case, to be sure, but it points up the depth of people's feelings about their looks and the joy that a successful rhinoplasty can deliver.

Margo is in her late teens and she is suffering from acute leukemia. While she is in chemotherapy and currently in remission, the long-range outlook for her life expectancy is not good, and she knows it. She also knows that great strides have been made in recent years in understanding this disease and that leukemia patients are living longer and longer. She is optimistic about a medical breakthrough and handles her illness with amazing courage and grace.

Margo and her parents came to see me some months ago because the dislike she had for her nose had, if anything, increased after she learned about her illness. "Given my shorter-than-average life expectancy," she told me, "I feel it's kind of urgent for me to have my nose fixed rather quickly, so that I can enjoy the rest of my life as a pretty girl, not a homely one."

Margo's parents told me that this was not a sudden decision on her part — she had, since she was thirteen, spoken about the possibility of improving her nose by means of plastic surgery. While they had never set a timetable for such an operation, they had not discouraged her about it, either. Now that she was determined to go ahead with it, they felt they should support her in this desire and they shared her expressed feeling that, if time was to be short, she should have the surgery soon.

There was nothing about Margo's looks that would tell you she had a serious illness. She was five-foot six-inches tall, well built, had auburn hair and bright flecks in her green eyes. Without ever having worn braces, her teeth were just about perfect. Her smile warmed the room. Given the circumstances, her cheerfulness was amazing. I booked her for summer surgery as she was just finishing her first year of college and would have a three-month vacation.

If any rhinoplasty operation can be said to be "simple," this one was. Margo had a prominent hump on an otherwise normal nose. I removed the hump, made the nose slightly shorter, and turned up the tip almost imperceptibly. Throughout the consultation period and surgical scheduling, I was in frequent touch with Margo's oncologist, who had wholeheartedly agreed to the rhinoplasty. He felt that there was no medical contraindication for the operation.

Four months have gone by since Margo's surgery, and the swelling is just about gone. Margo is lovely looking — truly. Her face matches her disposition, which is, more than ever, warm, sunny, and optimistic. She chose not to return to college this year, wanting to be near her family and her doctor. She is working in a clothing store, which she says she loves, but plans to return to college next year if her health permits it. She is still in remission.

"I can't tell you," she said to me a few days ago, "how my new nose has affected my outlook on everything. Do you find it strange that I have a serious illness and yet I'm happy? I am, you know — it's just heavenly to look in the mirror and see this nice nose. Maybe it's crazy, but I kind of feel it's given me a new lease on life. I think I'm going to make it. And I'm glad I'm going to make it with a pretty face."

Margo's parents tell me that, despite the cloud that hangs over her, she is almost always cheerful. She has made new friends at work, sees a great deal of her old high school classmates, and is dating an exchange student from Belgium. "We know," says Margo's father, "that it was one hundred percent right to let her have that nose operation. We loved her with the bump on her nose and we love her now. We haven't changed. But she has. It seems she loves herself a lot more now that she has a face that appeals to her. We're just going to go on hoping. . . ."

I don't know if there are a great number of guys who get their noses fixed, unless it's because of some football accident or something. But I had mine done because it was long and hooked over and I thought I looked like Ernie in "The Muppets," sort of with a grappling hook where my nose was supposed to be.

Anyway, my girlfriend had her nose fixed, though I didn't think her old nose was at all bad, and it made her very happy. She talked to me about my having an operation and, to my surprise, my parents weren't at all upset at the idea. My mother, in particular, was all for it.

My parents went to the doctor with me when I got out of high school and it was quite a few months before he could schedule it, which wasn't the worst because I could have time to change my mind if I wanted to. But the closer I came to it, the more certain I was that it was a good idea. I had really hated my nose for years.

I think it came out neat. It doesn't bend forward anymore. It's straight, as you can see, very masculine, I think. I helped to pay for it myself with my cash graduation gifts, and I had worked after school and saved some of my salary. But my parents paid most of it. My dad kids me now about my good looks, but I don't mind. I like to look in the mirror when I shave. I didn't use to. Let's face it: I'm much better looking.

The speaker at our high school graduation told us, "Be everything that you can be." I buy that. If I can improve my appearance in any way, why shouldn't I?

"The horror of that moment," the King went on, "I shall never, *never* forget!"

"You will, though," the Queen said, "if you don't make a memorandum of it."

— LEWIS CARROLL, *Through the Looking-Glass*

Chemabrasion and Dermabrasion | 9

YEARS AGO, I WAS A PROFESSIONAL dancer and quite successful, too. I performed all over this country, and abroad as well. In recent years, however, my life has been hard and painful. As I grew too old to dance professionally, I tried a new career as a photographer, but was unsuccessful in that endeavor. Five years ago I was divorced, and two years ago my only daughter was stricken with a serious and disabling illness. At that time, fifty-five years old, I sought psychiatric help because I was so depressed.

I had never thought of myself as being beautiful; I wasn't. But I always thought of myself as attractive, and even today people tell me I have a dancer's body and that my carriage is typical of people who have spent years training for the stage. My eyes are dark, my hair hasn't turned gray at all, and, for the most part, my looks are what you would expect for someone my age. But my skin started to wrinkle early, particularly on my cheekbones and above my lip. I also developed puffy eyelid bags under my eyes.

Last year, I had several consultations with a plastic surgeon, and he thought that a blepharoplasty operation, followed by a chemical peel in the wrinkled areas, might improve my appearance. At that time, my self-confidence was at an all-time low and I was hopeful that an improvement in my looks would give me back some of my confidence.

I had the eye operation in January and the chemabrasion in May.

I faced both procedures with a mixture of fear and anticipation. There was more fear before the eyelid operation; by the time I had the chemabrasion, I knew that cosmetic surgery wasn't a bad experience at all. Now that both operations are a thing of the past, I'm happy that I thought of cosmetic surgery in the first place. I think my self-esteem had been shattered by the events in my life and now I've been able to get back some of it.

My sister and I have opened a dance school for children, and the business is going well. The combination of a change in my appearance and of working again without being unhappy every time I look in the mirror has helped me to cope better with misfortune when she visits me. I am ever so much more optimistic. I know the future is going to be better than the recent past. I see my life as full of new opportunities.

No matter how careful we are, the human skin inevitably loses some of its smooth texture: it wrinkles, it sags, and unwelcome patches of pigmentation may appear. As with all aspects of our looks and appearance, a great deal depends upon our genes. However, certain other factors lend a hand to nature as she takes her toll in the aging process. Chief among these factors is that self-inflicted offense: excessive exposure of the skin to the sun.

Many of us believe that a "healthy" tan imparts a feeling of well-being, reinforced every time we look in the mirror and see our tanned countenance. As friends admire the tan, this feeling of well-being is again reaffirmed, along with the irrepressible adage: *you can't be too thin, too rich, or too tan.* (Remember how healthy John Kennedy looked with his Palm Beach tan, compared to Richard Nixon's pallor, when they had their famous TV debate? Many historians believe this perception of a healthy candidate clinched the election for J.F.K.)

Unfortunately, the long-range outlook for those who spend a great deal of time in the sun, unprotected by hat or lotion, is not favorable: excessive sun triggers degenerative changes in the skin, irregular pigmentation, and precancerous (sometimes even cancerous, as Ronald Reagan can testify) lesions. All this is in addition to premature wrinkling and loss of elasticity of the skin.

Incidentally, the jury is still out on the new, so-called safe suntan parlors that have sprung up all over the nation. These new sunlamps are said to filter out the dangerous rays in the ultraviolet spectrum, thereby making it possible for tanning to take place without the danger of inducing skin cancer. Their safety has not yet been definitely established. In fact, many physicians are puzzled by the Federal Food and Drug Administration's lack of regulation of these suntanning machines.

Even for people who are quite careful about exposure to the sun — and, I should add, the wind, another, if lesser, offender — a time comes when wrinkles and pouches make their appearance on the face and the skin loses its smooth feel as well as some of its elasticity. But there is good news: until a relatively short time ago, one had to accept these signs of aging or try to disguise them with makeup; now they can be considerably diminished by certain cosmetic surgery procedures. We already examined what a facelift and eyelid surgery can do. Chemabrasion and dermabrasion are two other procedures growing in popularity due to the improvements in technique during the last three decades and the number of skilled and trained physicians qualified to perform these delicate procedures.

Chemabrasion vs. Dermabrasion

The skin is a many-layered structure. Both chemabrasion, which peels away the top layer of the skin with a chemical solution, and dermabrasion, which grinds it away with a mechanical instrument (a rotating wheel), decrease facial wrinkles by making it possible for a new, healthy outer layer of unwrinkled skin to grow where the old, damaged one has been removed.

There is not a general consensus in the medical profession about which procedure is "better"; nor even which one is better for certain skin conditions. Some doctors who work with both techniques believe that many of the conditions that bring patients to a consulting room — superficial pigmentation, fine wrinkles like the vertical lines of the upper lip or crisscross wrinkles on the cheeks, superficial skin lesions resulting from excessive exposure to the sun, and many types of elevated scars and blemishes — can be treated with equal effectiveness by either technique. However, doctors experienced in both tend to favor dermabrasion for the treatment of acne scars and chemabrasion (often referred to as a "chemical peel") for wrinkles.

The world-renowned dermatologist Dr. Norman Orentreich of New York prefers dermabrasion to chemabrasion for most conditions, including the small wrinkles near the eye known as *rhytides*. He believes that, by and large, the results he obtains from dermabrasion are superior to those from chemabrasion. He also considers the mechanical technique of dermabrasion, over which he can exercise control, to be safer than the chemical peel process, in which it is difficult to predict how an individual's skin will respond to a given chemical.

My own preference, and one shared by most plastic surgeons, is for chemical peeling for the reduction or elimination of fine lines and wrinkles of the face. I believe the results are superior to those obtained by mechanical abrasion. I also prefer peeling for the treatment of some forms of abnormal pigmentation, particularly of the eyelids, since the use of a mechanical instrument so close to the eye is worrisome. On the other hand, it has been my experience that dermabrasion is more effective for the treatment of acne scars, small raised scars of the skin, and smoothing surface irregularities resulting from incisions made in previous, noncosmetic surgery.

It is wise to carefully consider the preference of the doctor (or doctors) you consult. Then, depending on what makes sense to you in terms of your particular problem, and also upon which doctor you want to treat you, the decision will be yours to make.

Chemabrasion (Chemical Peeling)

I mentioned earlier that the skin is a many-layered structure. The top layer is called the *epidermis*; beneath it lies the *dermis*, containing fibrous connective tissue; below that, a layer of fat. Chemabrasion, or chemical peeling (also called chemosurgery), is a controlled burning of the skin in which a caustic chemical, usually *phenol*, is skillfully applied in order to remove the epidermis and part of the dermis. After the chemical application, and for some days beyond that, the old skin remains in place until a new skin has formed underneath it. This is in contrast to dermabrasion, in which the top layer of the skin is actually removed during the procedure.

The results of a chemical peeling, when full healing has taken place, can be truly dramatic. The face will appear to be firmer.

Wrinkles will be eliminated or diminished to a great degree. Although the skin's elasticity, once it is gone, cannot be restored, the texture of the skin after chemabrasion will be considerably improved.

How Chemabrasion Developed

The origin of chemabrasion as part of modern-day medicine reads like a detective story. Peeling of the skin with chemicals began many decades ago as a nonmedical treatment administered by lay operators, probably in eastern Europe. The technique found its way to the United States shortly after World War II, when clinics for skin peeling were set up, the first ones in Florida and California. These clinics were not under any government or medical regulations or supervision.

Rumors of the benefits of skin peeling caught the attention of dermatologists and plastic surgeons. Little reliable information could be obtained, however, since no scientific reports were being published. We do know that responsible plastic surgeons, such as Sir Harold Gillies, known as the father of modern plastic surgery, were aware of chemical skin peeling as early as the 1930s, and that these doctors dabbled in the procedure. They did not develop it significantly, however, or advocate its use for aesthetic improvement of facial skin.

By the 1950s, face-peeling "parlors" and clinics had been established in more than half the states, many in Sunbelt areas where exposure to the sun increases the percentage of the population suffering from premature wrinkling and abnormal pigmentation. In that decade, reputable surgeons such as Dr. Thomas Baker of Miami, Florida, began an investigation to determine what the chemical components were that made up the mix being used. Researchers visited some of the peeling parlors, with investigators posing as potential patients, so that their requests for information — not otherwise forthcoming — would be considered natural. Despite the lay operators' efforts to protect their secret formulas, perseverance won out. Dr. Baker finally obtained the phenol formula that is still widely in use.

The formula, which evolved out of trial and error, makes little scientific sense because some of its components are not chemically compatible. Nonetheless, it works, and the medical profession continues to use it because it is effective and reasonably safe. There are other chemicals that are also used in chemabrasion, including *trichloracetic* and *bichloracetic* acids. Much discussion and some controversy has occurred over which of these mixtures is most effective, although there is little discernible difference in the results achieved by these various chemicals.

Indications for Chemabrasion

Chemabrasion is carried out to eradicate or improve shallow wrinkles and creases, fine lines about the eyes and the lips, minor skin blemishes, as well as abnormal pigmentation. It is not useful in removing pouches or lifting a sagging skin. Other procedures — eyelid surgery and a facelift, for example — are the treatments of choice for those conditions.

Sometimes the chemical peel will be done in conjunction with a facelift if only small skin areas, such as the lips or forehead, are involved. Treatment of larger areas, however, or a complete facial peeling cannot be done at the same time as a facelift. On page 53 I explained how the facelift operation involves a virtual lifting away of the skin from the deeper tissues of the face. Adding a chemical burn to the skin at the same time could compromise the blood supply upon which successful healing is so dependent. Even beyond this, the strain on the patient could be too much, the procedure too lengthy, and the recovery period a bit complicated.

In cases where both a facelift and a full-face chemical peel are planned, the peel should be deferred for at least three weeks after the first procedure, to allow the skin to recover from that surgery. However, if fine wrinkling of the facial skin is the primary problem, and jowls, double chin, and sagging skin of the cheeks and neck are the secondary problem, it is often advisable to perform the face peel first, followed by a face- and neck-lift three or more weeks later. Sometimes, the result of the peel is so successful that the facelift surgery is postponed indefinitely.

Chemabrasion can also be highly successful in people with marked horizontal wrinkling of the forehead skin, if they have not yet developed deep vertical frown lines, or ptosis (dropping) of the brows. A peel of the entire forehead is performed as a unit and can be carried out with or without a full face peel. And, while I said that a complete face peeling cannot be performed at the same time as a facelift, a forehead peel *can* be done at the same time.

At times, chemabrasion is also recommended for the treatment of many superficial skin blemishes such as patchy pigmentation, multiple keratoses (benign pigmented elevations of the skin), and "spiderweb" blood vessels. For such problems, chemical peel can offer a prolonged, sometimes permanent, solution.

One of the most common reasons that middle-aged people — almost always women — see a plastic surgeon or dermatologist is because they are unhappy about the vertical lines that develop on their lips, especially the upper lip. The major complaint is that their lipstick "runs" into these lines. This problem often starts in the early forties, although many women do not develop such lines until they are in their fifties (again, genes are at work). Since men can always grow a mustache, they are rarely troubled by this problem. Lip lines are probably unrelated to cigarette smoking, since they occur with equal frequency in nonsmokers.

While lip lines are one of the first signs of aging (along with puffs or bags of the eyelids), the lip can be peeled at any age. One need not wait for a facelift or eyelid surgery to have chemabrasion performed on such a limited area. It can be done at any time.

Good Candidates for Chemabrasion

The ideal candidates for a full-face chemical peel are usually in middle age and have dry skin which has been abused with repeated exposure to the elements, particularly solar rays. Many interwoven, very fine wrinkles of the facial skin are present, frequently accompanied by blemishes, pigmented spots, and small broken blood vessels.

Such patients are often of northern European descent, with a typically fair-skinned Scandinavian or Scotch-Irish complexion and light-colored eyes and hair. Their skin is usually dry to begin with and repeated exposure to the sun succeeds in drying it out altogether. As the natural oils disappear, there is little or no protection against wrinkling. In some patients, such excessive wrinkling is hereditary. Very rarely, we find it is related to a pituitary disorder.

A person with the type of complexion I've just described is, as a matter of fact, the better candidate for chemical peeling than someone with an olive complexion. A more pigmented skin tends to show a line of demarcation between the treated and untreated areas. Since the treated part will remain light in color for a long time, if not permanently, the contrast is less marked in fair-skinned people. Dark-complected people also have a tendency to blotchiness in both the treated and untreated areas. Chemabrasion is not advisable for blacks because the treated areas will never again match the rest of the facial skin.

While minor skin blemishes are amenable to improvement with chemabrasion, birthmarks, particularly if they are large, cannot be eliminated with this process. Chemosurgery on parts of the body other than the face must be approached with great caution. The skin of the neck, hands, and body is not nearly as rich in sweat glands and hair follicles as is the facial skin. These glands and follicles are referred to as "skin appendages," and it is their presence that ensures prompt and safe healing of the skin after chemical peel or dermabrasion, since the regrowth of new skin cells to cover the abraded area originates *within* these skin appendages. Areas where the appendages are relatively sparse, such as the neck and back of the hands, are apt to heal more slowly, sometimes with problems developing during the healing process.

The skin of the neck is also very thin, and it is difficult to control the depth of the burn from the chemical used in a chemabrasion procedure. In fact, use of this procedure on arms, hands, or the chest has not often been crowned with success — certainly not the success one can look forward to with chemical peeling of the face. When hand peeling is done, the hands must be kept out of water for a minimum of five to seven days, or scarring and overpigmentation may result. I, for one, do not do chemabrasion on the hands. I do not believe the results warrant it.

On the other hand, the most dramatic changes in a person's appearance are those brought about by a full face peel in a highly suitable candidate. A heavily wrinkled person, particularly a woman, can actually look as much, if not more than, a decade older than her true age. When such wrinkling exists, a facelift, even an extensive one, cannot eliminate this aged look; but a chemical peel can work wonders, sometimes a near-miracle. One of my patients, a woman of fifty-one who looked like she was seventy years old when she first walked into my office, was unaware that chemical peeling existed as a branch of cosmetic surgery.

Doris was a fine painter who lived on Cape Cod and spent a good deal of her free time at her hobby: big-game fishing. She was extremely weather-beaten; her wrinkled face and the blotchy pigmentation of the skin on the backs of her hands made her look like the old woman of the sea. But her trim figure, athletic walk, natural, soft hair, and youthful manner of dressing identified her as being much younger than her face indicated.

I noted the quick smile and warm personality of this half-young, half-aged woman as she told me that she looked twenty years older than her husband and more like a grandmother to her children than their mother. At first she told me that she had accepted what fate had handed her. Then, suddenly bursting into tears, she told me that once, while changing clothes in the locker room of her club, she had overheard two acquaintances comparing her wrinkled face to that of Margo, the fictitious heroine in *Lost Horizon*, who, returning to her home after a period of living in Shangri-la, where no one ever grows old, finds herself aged and wrinkled. Doris had been terribly hurt by this and grew determined to do something about it. She asked me what I thought a facelift could do for her.

She was quite dismayed when I said that a facelift would do very little for her particular skin. I then proceeded to tell her about chemabrasion and how it might make a significant difference in her case. She was amazed. I told her as much as I could about the procedure and gave her some literature to take home and read. She did quite a bit of research on chemical peeling and when I next saw her for a follow-up consultation, she had grown remarkably sophisticated about the technique. She said she wanted to be booked for the operation, and I agreed with her, since she was an ideal candidate for it.

It all went extremely well. Indeed, the result was so astounding and startling that at first even some of her friends didn't recognize her.

"To think," she told me when she had completely recovered from the surgery, "that a year ago I had never heard the word *chemabrasion*. It's all been like a miracle. My skin looks younger and feels softer; all those wrinkles are gone from my cheeks and my lip. I feel as though I've been given another start in life. Now I think I look like the character Margo in *Lost Horizon* before she left that never-never land of Shangri-la where people didn't age. And you know who's happiest? *My children.* One of them said, 'Hey! I've got the prettiest mom on the block!' "

Not all patients, of course, enjoy such outstanding results. One of the difficulties with the peeling process is that the results vary a great deal from person to person and it is not possible to determine exactly how effective a peel will be. Anyone who tells you otherwise is misleading you.

While spot or area peeling, such as that done on the upper lip, the chin, the forehead, and sometimes even the lower eyelids, are commonly done (the upper lip is the site treated most frequently by this technique), chemical peeling of the entire face is an infrequent procedure. The number of such peels done also varies with geography. Full-face peels are rare in the northern part of the United States; Florida and other Sunbelt states, with a greater number of older people and people who have had more extensive sun exposure, lead the country in the number of such procedures performed annually.

Chemical peeling is very popular in Hollywood and Beverly Hills. A number of new "peeling parlors," run by operators with no medical training whatsoever, have sprung up in southern California. This is an unfortunate development, because it coincides with a trend among quite young women to undergo a full-face peel in the belief that such a peel will delay the need for a facelift in years to come. I don't know how this belief sprang up or why it caught on so rapidly in southern California. The truth is that a deep skin peel will permanently mar the color and texture of their skin.

BEFORE THE SURGERY

Photographs   As with all cosmetic surgery, preoperative photographs are required so the surgeon can determine exactly what areas he will work in, and how much needs to be done in each spot.

Medical history

A detailed medical history is taken before chemabrasion is scheduled because certain health conditions preclude chemical face peeling. Foremost among these is chronic renal (kidney) disease, in which the function of the kidneys is impaired. Liver disease such as hepatitis and cirrhosis are also contraindications for this procedure because the caustic chemical used can be harmful to people suffering these ailments. Here's why: minute amounts of the chemical substance (usually phenol) are absorbed into the system during face peeling and then excreted by the kidneys after first undergoing some chemical alterations in the liver. An ailing liver or kidney might have trouble altering and disposing of the caustic chemical.

Various cardiac arrhythmias have been reported during deep phenol face peeling. To my knowledge, none has proven to have a serious consequence and all have been of very short duration. However, because of these reports, many surgeons prefer to monitor the patient's heart with continuous EKG during the operation. In fact, the whole subject of this procedure is controversial — deep, *full*-face peel, that is — and most of us exercise caution in evaluating candidates for it, as well as caution in performing the procedure.

Hospital stay

Chemabrasion can be performed either in a hospital or on an ambulatory basis, depending on how much peeling will be done. If a small area is to be treated, such as the lip, a patient can go home the same day. Most doctors favor a hospital stay for a full-face peel. The usual stay is one to three days, with admission the day before the procedure so that routine examinations and laboratory tests can be carried out. Should you enter the hospital for this procedure, you will be told to wash your face thoroughly with an antibacterial soap the night before and the morning of the surgery.

Anesthesia General anesthesia is not required for chemabrasion, but adequate sedation is administered, usually intravenously, before and during the surgery. Both tranquilizers and painkillers are used in sufficient amounts so that there is no significant discomfort beyond a burning sensation for a few seconds, or perhaps a minute or two, when the chemical is applied. General anesthesia is an option for those who want it.

The Technique

Before the operation your face will be cleansed with ether or a similar skin degreaser to remove any skin oils or soap that may have remained on your skin. The phenol compound is then applied with a brush or an applicator. You will feel a momentary stinging or burning sensation, but it will pass quickly.

The skin is gently stretched during the application so the treated area gets an even coating with the chemical. You will not see it, of course, but the skin will first turn frosty white. Some swelling will follow, and the color will then change to a deep red blush.

The procedure is carried out section by section. In order to avoid a visible demarcation line between the treated and the untreated skin in a full-face peel, the chemical application goes slightly above the hairline (no permanent damage is done to the hair) and just below the jawline. The chemical will go right to the bright red border of the lips, which may result in some blistering, but it's done that way to prevent a thin band of untreated skin being visible after recovery.

After each section is treated, it is covered by waterproof adhesive tape that leaves only the eyes, lips, and nostrils exposed. The tape improves the final result by continuing the active chemical ingredients of the application and preventing their evaporation. The tape is not particularly comfortable, but it's removed after forty-eight hours — usually followed by a sigh of relief. There is some controversy over whether taping is essential in deep peeling. It seems to promote a deeper peel, and therefore is more effective in the removal of the wrinkles. When the surgeon does a more superficial peel, the tape is sometimes not applied. Nor will it be used on patients with very sensitive skin.

I would like to tell you a bit more about the chemical used in this procedure. Phenol, the most commonly used substance, is in a solution with distilled water, croton oil, and liquid soap. The croton oil serves as an additional irritant. The solution "burns" the skin, destroying its superficial layers. The burning does not penetrate the full thickness of the skin, the depth of penetration being largely determined by the amount of the solution applied and the concentration or strength of the mixture.

Oddly enough, we learned many years ago that the depth of burning was more easily controlled by using a highly concentrated solution because it does not penetrate as deeply as a weak one. Untrained people think that diluting the phenol will weaken it and make it safer to use, when actually the opposite is true. Strong solutions literally "coagulate" the superficial skin layers, which then act as a barrier to any deeper penetration. Weaker solutions burn at a less intense rate and can continue to penetrate the skin, seeping into the system. Because small amounts of the chemicals are always absorbed into the body, the entire procedure is carried out with a deliberate degree of slowness in order to allow the body to cope with the absorption.

When the solution is applied to the face, there is the momentary stinging I mentioned. But phenol actually anesthetizes the nerve endings, and the amount of sedation and painkiller the surgeon injects is sufficient to make this transient pain tolerable. The discomfort experienced is, of course, directly proportional to each person's pain threshold, which varies greatly, person to person.

AFTER THE SURGERY

Pain and itching   After chemabrasion, patients have a variety of symptoms, mostly unpleasant but all bearable, particularly if you dwell more on the great improvements that can be anticipated after recovery. These symptoms are related to the surface scab that forms, and include a sensation of tightness, or being confined (claustrophobics beware!), of warmth, pain, and — later on in the convalescent period — itching. The scab formation limits facial movement, and for many people, this is an uncomfortable feeling. The itching is related to the healing process going on beneath the scab. It can be quite intense during the first few days or until the scab separates, at which time it subsides rapidly. In perhaps 2 percent of all chemabrasion patients, the itching can persist for several weeks, although there are a few drugs that can be prescribed (for some, but not all, patients) to alleviate it.

Speaking, eating   If the peel included the lips, it is not advisable to speak for the first forty-eight hours, during which time your diet is restricted to liquids taken through a straw. Bed rest is recommended for the first twenty-four hours postoperatively; forty-eight hours if a large area of your face was treated.

Removal of the mask   When the adhesive mask is removed, the skin's surface is dusted with a medicated powder, producing a thin, coagulated surface. For the next three days, you will reapply the powder several times a day. Although your diet will be liberalized at this point, both chewing and talking must still be kept to a minimum. Mild, general activities are permissible, but overexertion and anything that causes sweating should be avoided.

Formation of the new skin

By the third day, the swelling begins to subside and dry crusts start to form, much like those you had as a child when you "skinned" your knee in a fall on a cement walk. These crusts begin to loosen, and seven to ten days after surgery, they separate and fall off, leaving a layer beneath that heals by the spread of epithelial cells to form a new skin. All the crusts are usually off after two weeks. However, they should not be forced or picked off; they will let you know when they're ready to go.

Medication and ointments

On the fifth day after the removal of the adhesive mask (seven days after surgery), a liberal coating of a bland cold cream or a prescribed ointment must be applied to the whole treated surface. Different doctors favor different medications and ointments. Vitamin E ointment, antibiotic ointments, bland creams, and powders all have their advocates. I doubt that it makes much difference which is used. In fact, to the consternation of Pablo Manzoni, the famous cosmetics expert, some surgeons even recommend the application of Crisco, a pure vegetable oil. What is important is that the wound heal as cleanly as possible and without infection, since that would cause the wounding to go deeper and could result in a scar.

The day following the application of the cream, the powdery mask is easily removed, revealing a delicate pink new skin. After that, the face can be washed daily with mild soap and water and patted dry. The new skin should be kept moist with cold cream or a moisturizer.

Makeup

After one more week, light makeup may be applied. Two to three weeks after the powdery mask comes off, it is all right to use regular makeup.

Different postsurgical treatments

Your physician may prescribe a postsurgical treatment different from the one I have described; there is considerable difference of opinion between doctors as to how the scab should be managed. While many prefer the scabbing over and crusting technique, there are others who recommend the immediate application of antibiotic creams to the treated area of skin, commencing at once after the application of the peel solution. They try to avoid the hard crust stage. I do not believe there is very much, if any, difference in the end result, and I certainly recommend that you follow the advice of your own doctor, whatever it might be.

The period of convalescence

Because you will not be looking very presentable, you're going to be house-bound for a week to ten days. This is one guarantee I *can* give you: you won't want to see your friends during this period. You may not even want to see certain members of your family. Certainly until the scab separates and the new skin is revealed, you will look far from attractive if you've had a full-face peel; you won't look terrific even if you had a partial peel. Some people also have a good deal of swelling. I am telling you all this, not to scare you away from chemabrasion, but to prepare you psychologically for what the mirror will show you during your early days of convalescence.

When the new skin arrives

The newly healed skin can be expected to look bright pink in color at first, and though this intense pink will fade rapidly, some such coloration will remain. It fades gradually over a period of several months, although eight to ten months is not out of the realm of possibility. It will end as a pale patch of skin, distinctly paler than the surrounding skin and usually without blemishes, blotches, or pigmentation. The paleness is more obvious when the peel is only on one area of the face, such as the upper lip, particularly if the untreated surrounding skin has freckles, pigment spots, or blotches. The difference is permanent and requires makeup, although such covering can be minimal.

Chemical skin peeling can be repeated, but not before a rest period of at least a year. This is rarely called for, although someone who has had one area of the face peeled and is satisfied with the results will frequently request a second peel on another facial area.

DERMABRASION (SKIN PLANING)

Dermabrasion, also known as skin planing, is a process which removes the superficial layers of the skin by mechanically scraping or grinding them away. It is effective in reducing the number of fine wrinkles and in improving the appearance of skin scarred and pitted by acne, as well as removing some freckles and pigmentation. It is a delicate operation and calls for considerable skill and experience.

This procedure was originally accomplished with sandpaper, literally. During World War II, dermabrasion was performed to remove dirt or fragments of metal embedded in the skin following blast injuries, and in the late forties, to remove skin tattoos.

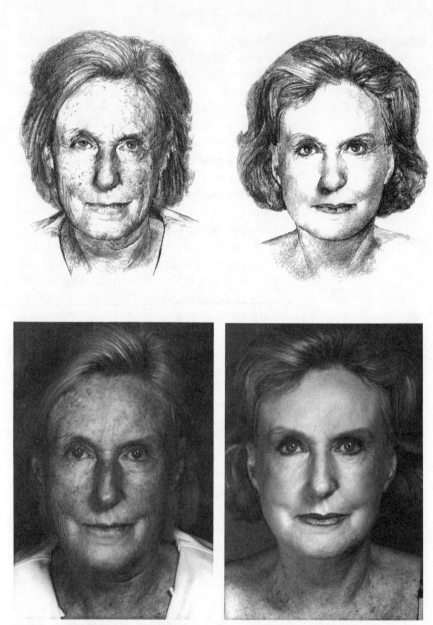

Finely wrinkled skin made this woman an ideal candidate for a facelift combined with chemabrasion. Dermabrasion could have been used instead of chemabrasion.

Dermabrasion has grown much more sophisticated since then.

The use, in the forties, of an electrically driven cylinder wrapped in abrasive paper was followed by the development of the rough wire brush and the burr impregnated with diamond particles, both of which are used today for dermabrasion. Either of these is attached to a motor or air-driven cable that revolves at high speeds and abrades the skin's surface to grind off the top layers. The speed of revolution is adjustable and under the control of the operator. Nature, with a bit of outside help, then resurfaces the face. This technique can be compared to a gravel or brush burn. At some time when you were a child, you must have fallen from a bicycle or onto the floor of the school gym and scraped your knee or elbow. Remember the tight scab that formed and how the scab separated in a few days, revealing fresh, red, new skin beneath? That is exactly what occurs during dermabrasion.

The degree of improvement of the face after dermabrasion varies and depends on the type of blemishes and the depth with which they were embedded in the skin. Some faces are improved enormously, and the results are most gratifying to patient and doctor alike. Where there is deeper scarring and only marginal improvement, a second and even a third procedure may be necessary. In such cases, there is a wait of at least half a year — a full year is better — before the procedure can be repeated.

Acne Scars and Dermabrasion

Dermabrasion is usually the procedure of choice to improve scarring due to acne. Such scars can be visualized as small craters on the skin. The base (or bottom) of the crater is thick scar tissue, while the edge (or perimeter) of the crater is heaped-up scar tissue covered by layers of cells (the *epithelium*) and raised from the surrounding skin. While mechanical grinding of these crater edges is more efficient than the burn peel process, it is usually impossible to grind away the skin so deeply that the bottom of the crater is removed. To do so would destroy the entire thickness of the skin and result in additional scarring.

While dermabrasion during active infection has not proven hazardous to the healing process, it is preferable to perform the operation when the acne problem has subsided.

In dermabrading acne scars, no result is 100 percent perfect, but, depending on the depth and nature of the scars, abrasions subsequent to the first one can continue to improve the condition. People who have been unhappy about their acne and the scars that remained are usually extremely pleased with any improvement that can be made.

Joanne, a kindergarten teacher in her mid-twenties, came to see me about having a bump removed from her nose. She told me she was enthusiastic about cosmetic surgery because she had suffered from bad acne, which had left her face noticeably scarred, and a Boston dermatologist had "performed miracles" (her words) with dermabrasion. "You can see," she said, "that there are still traces of the acne scars but, believe me, doctor, this is nothing compared to the way they were three years ago.

"I was extremely self-conscious," Joanne continued, "and from the time I was in high school until I was twenty-one, I hardly ever dated. I thought I looked a mess, although I was probably more aware of the acne first, and then those scars, than other people might have been when they looked at me. It totally destroyed my self-esteem. In fact, I was so withdrawn that I almost didn't go to college. But I was accepted at Radcliffe and decided to go. Incidentally, I was graduated in the top ten in my class.

"At twenty-two, I decided that before I went to interview for a job, I was going to find out if something could be done about the scars on my face. I went to my former pediatrician, and he suggested I see a dermatologist. He gave me the name of the man who did the dermabrasion several months later.

"It turned around my life. I have a good job doing what I want to do, working with children, and I'm dating quite a bit these days. But now I would like to improve my nose if it's possible. I found out something about myself: looks may not be the most important thing in the world, but it's certainly great for my ego to like what I see in the mirror."

Some acne scars are very deep, resembling ice-pick wounds. These can only be superficially improved by dermabrasion. Recently, a technique has been employed which, along with dermabrasion, offers patients more opportunity to be helped. The deep pits, together with a small circumference of surrounding skin, are removed with a small, round punch. This punched-out area is replaced with a small graft taken with the same-sized punch from behind the ear. Healing occurs with a small round scar. Patients who have had this procedure find it a good trade-off: the deep ice-pick scar has been traded for a flatter one that is much softer in appearance.

There is no age limit for dermabrasion — upper or lower — for this surgical procedure can be done at all ages. However, the older the person, the longer will it take for the skin to heal.

BEFORE THE SURGERY

Photographs   Preoperative photographs will be needed by your physician so that he can examine closely the areas of your face to be worked on. He will either take these pictures himself or send you to a medical photographer. Some doctors require only black-and-white photos; others prefer to see the pictures in both black-and-white and color.

Medical history   It is essential, as with chemabrasion, that a full medical history be obtained by the doctor, and this will probably include information about drug sensitivities as well as information on whether there was prior chemabrasion or dermabrasion done on your face. If you recently had a skin rash or an outbreak of herpes, be sure to report it to your doctor.

The evening before surgery   The evening before the operation, your hair should be shampooed thoroughly. Men are asked to shave closely the day that the surgery is performed.

Hospital stay   This surgery is usually performed by trained dermatologists and plastic surgeons. Some operate in their offices, using local anesthesia. Others prefer to do the procedure in the hospital, in which case the patient is discharged the next day.

Anesthesia — When a full-face peel is involved, many surgeons prefer a general anesthesia. When the choice is for a local, an anesthetic such as Xylocaine or Novocain is injected under the skin, after administering adequate sedation. Some doctors, especially dermatologists, prefer to freeze the skin, literally, until it assumes a boardlike quality which, because of its stability, facilitates the abrading. The skin can be frozen by spraying it with ethyl chloride or applying freon freeze packs directly to the surface. In any case, either the patient or the skin must be anesthetized, since the pain of abrasion would be quite severe without it.

The Technique

The face can be abraded completely in a single session, or the doctor and patient may agree upon doing it in several sessions, debrading one area at a time.

Bit by bit, the surgeon grinds away the superficial skin until he reaches the desired level. To stem the bleeding after the procedure, warm air from a hair dryer is blown over the abraded area. This also helps in forming a thick incrustation over the surface. Some surgeons then apply an antibiotic ointment and a dressing; others do not. If used, the dressing is removed the next day.

The entire procedure takes from a half-hour to an hour for a full-face dermabrasion, proportionately less for smaller areas.

Just as in chemical abrasion, a crust forms over the entire abraded surface immediately following dermabrasion. This crust is the body's attempt to protect itself and to wall off the injured area of skin so that body fluids are not lost and healing can take place. New skin cells are stimulated to grow as a result of the wounding process. These cells spread out from the many appendages (glands and hair follicles) deep within the skin. They proliferate and grow in a coalescing sheet beneath the crust, where an entirely new skin surface is formed. The crust, having served its protective purpose, is then shed. Without the presence of infection, this process of new skin-cell growth, which is called *epithelialization*, is complete in about ten days.

Success of the dermabrasion procedure depends upon this ability of the deeper layers of the skin to form this new surface epithelium and, except for special cases (where there have been bad burns or irradiation injuries), healing usually follows a normal regenerative course.

AFTER THE SURGERY

The first days after surgery

If you go into the hospital for a dermabrasion procedure, you will, as I said, be discharged the day following surgery. If the surgery is done on an ambulatory basis, you will go home the same day, probably a few hours after the procedure is completed.

Quite likely, your doctor will instruct you to use a warm hair dryer for the first day or so to maintain and keep dry the superficial crusting.

You will be given some pain medication and possibly a sleeping pill or two. Antibiotics are not strictly necessary, although some doctors do prescribe them.

When the crust begins to form, it could develop near your mouth, making it difficult to open it. A liquid diet will help — in fact, you probably would not be able to open your mouth sufficiently to chew solid food. After the third day, the swelling, which is normal and to be expected, will begin to subside and, as that happens, you'll start to feel more comfortable.

Shampoos, shaving

Daily use of cold creams or other bland ointments will help keep the crusts soft, but, until they separate from the skin in seven to ten days, shaving is not permitted. You can shampoo your hair, but with great caution, to avoid getting water or soap on your crusted face. In about two weeks, most normal activities can be resumed.

Sun protection   For the first three or four weeks after dermabrasion, no pigment forms in the skin, so it is essential that the treated areas be totally protected from the sun during this period. For several months after that, a hat and total screen block are essential if there's any possibility of being in the direct sun, or even in the indirect glare of solar rays. (I'll talk a bit more about this later in this chapter.)

CHEMABRASION COMBINED WITH DERMABRASION

A combination of chemabrasion and dermabrasion is sometimes indicated: dermabrasion is performed for the scarred areas, chemabrasion for the thin, uninvolved border areas. In such cases, the areas that will receive the chemical peel are treated first, with the phenol solution applied well into the areas of scarring to insure a good overlap between the peeled area and the site to be abraded.

THE POSSIBILITY OF COMPLICATIONS FROM CHEMABRASION AND DERMABRASION

Since abrasion and peeling traumatize the skin, it is possible for complications to occur. Of all the procedures we do in the realm of aesthetic surgery, chemical abrasion is the most worrisome to the doctor, because we have only limited control over what we're doing. When I cut cleanly and sharply with a knife or scissors, I am in accurate control of the length and depth of the cut. Painting an acid solution on the skin or applying a rapidly rotating abrasive wheel to it is quite another matter. Although this rarely occurs, the possibility exists that the acid solution or revolving wheel can extend too deeply into the skin.

Yet, from a practical point of view, both of these procedures are amazingly benign and real problems are uncommon.

I have described how abrasion removes most of the superficial pigment from the outer skin layers and results in a paler skin. However, in some patients — particularly those on birth control pills, especially estrogen therapy, as well as those who violate the "no direct sun after surgery" rule — hyperpigmentation (an excess of pigment formation) can result. It is possible that such conditions are the result of the procedure irritating the pigment cells and sensitizing them so that they overreact to any stimulus, including solar rays. Strange as it may seem, excessive pigmentation is best treated by yet another peel or abrasion. In cases of minor hyperpigmentation, creams with bleaching agents can sometimes be helpful.

Some people are unhappy when they see a difference in color between the treated and untreated areas of the face after chemabrasion. This is not really a complication — merely something more likely to occur in people with darker complexions, although it can happen to anyone, to a minor or major degree.

Infections after this type of surgery are rare because of the rich blood supply in the face. Tiny whiteheads, however, often appear in the treated areas; they can be removed during an office visit and leave no scars.

Birthmarks may appear darker after a chemical peel, and some surgeons favor removal of large birthmarks before dermabrasion or a chemical peel is undertaken.

Postoperative reddening of the skin sometimes persists for weeks or even months. This is more of an annoyance than a complication, and occasionally a physician will prescribe a mild cortisone ointment to hasten the disappearance of this surgical aftermath. Such redness is particularly evident after drinking even a small amount of alcohol. Giving up liquor completely for weeks, or even months, postoperatively is a good idea.

Frequently after chemabrasion, the skin pores appear to be enlarged, but this disappears in time. Keloids (excessive growth of scar tissue) rarely develop, but when they do, injections with steroid compounds can soften them and possibly limit their growth.

Though I do want you to know about the possibility of these complications, I would like to emphasize that skin biopsy studies on people who have had chemabrasion or dermabrasion show that, after the passage of considerable time, no damage ensues. Follow-up studies also show that the desirable changes following these procedures are consistently good and apparently permanent. Satisfaction among patients is high, and many who have had one area of the face treated return for additional procedures on other parts of the face.

If your physician suggests chemabrasion or dermabrasion as the best method for improving your skin, carefully consider his recommendation. If you are in doubt, get a second opinion. I favor second opinions, particularly when a full-face peel seems indicated. Be sure you obtain these opinions from physicians with experience in this highly specialized field. Do not, under any circumstances, consult a nonprofessional employed by a commercial peeling parlor. Chemabrasion and dermabrasion are two among a number of treatment methods that highly trained and responsible physician-specialists can employ successfully in the interests of their patients. Don't think you are avoiding an operation by having your face peeled in a lay "clinic." The face they scar may be your own.

Debunking Some Myths

There are those who will tell you that chemical peeling is more dangerous than dermabrasion, or vice versa. As far as I can determine, these techniques are equally safe. Complications are rare, but can occur with equal frequency in both. In either procedure, the skin can be removed too deeply and result in an open wound. While it is a fact that absorption of some of the caustic chemical used in chemabrasion could affect the liver or the kidneys, I am unaware of any serious problem that ever resulted from this.

Many people also believe that chemabrasion can be used to treat wrinkles of the neck, body, or hands. With a few selected exceptions, the answer to this is no; it is too risky. Peeling is usually limited to the face because healing on that portion of the body is excellent due to the superb blood supply to the facial skin. In my opinion, treating the entire surface of the backs of the hands with chemabrasion is not advisable. However, spot peeling of brown marks is safe and acceptable.

A popular misconception is that dermabrasion is the better procedure for wrinkles. My experience, and that of my colleagues, is that the chemical peel is much more effective for this purpose.

Many of my potential patients express the mistaken belief that peeling and dermabrasion are preventive measures to stave off aging and that they are useful in toning up the skin of young adults. On the contrary, these treatments should only be considered when there is clear indication of a skin condition that would be improved by them.

Another myth is that once a chemical peel or skin planing has been done, it must be repeated at intervals. This is not so. One treatment usually suffices, especially in the case of severe wrinkling.

Perhaps this is wishful thinking, but many people believe that after one of these procedures, the skin will eventually regain its pretreatment color and texture. This is not the case. After a peel, in particular, the area treated will always be smoother and paler than the surrounding skin. Makeup to cover the differences may be permanently needed.

A face peel, says yet another myth, is easier and just as effective as a facelift. This is absolutely false. A face peel actually does something quite different from a facelift. It removes or diminishes wrinkles, and while it will tighten the skin, it will not tighten sagging jowls or necks. Furthermore, in most cases, a face peel is much more uncomfortable than a facelift. While the latter is relatively easy on the patient, a chemical peel can be uncomfortable.

The Sun and You

Because this is so important to your health and recovery after chemabrasion or dermabrasion, I would like to reemphasize the importance of avoiding direct sunlight after either of these procedures.

It is unrealistic in this day and age, when so many of us enjoy tennis, golf, jogging, and other outdoor sports, to forbid all exposure to the sun's rays. However, passive sunbathing — lying on the beach or at the pool and letting the sun bake you — is self-defeating. You simply have to give up sunbathing if you wish cosmetic surgery to be effective. By following a few sensible rules, you can still live a reasonable outdoor life.

One absolute *must* after either procedure is to avoid direct sunlight. The new skin is depigmented; it has been stripped of its protective pigment layer. For my patients, I forbid direct sun exposure for eight to ten months after the surgery, depending on how fair the person's skin is. Out-and-out sunbathing is forbidden *forever*.

You should always have two types of protective sunning products on hand: a total sunblock cream (No. 15); and a good sunscreen (Nos. 10 through 15). Several years ago, the U.S. government imposed a rating system on the manufacturers of suntan lotions and creams: the number on the box, bottle, or label will tell you how effective the blocking agent is. The lower the number, the less protection you get. Numbers 2, 4, and 6 block out the least amount of ultraviolet rays; numbers 10 through 14 do a good job of blocking out the burning rays; a number 15 product is a "total block" or "superblock" agent and will protect you from all the harmful rays — provided you reapply the cream or lotion after each time you are in the water.

Once you have had a face peel or abrasion, you should never again permit yourself to be in the direct or indirect glare of the sun with less than a No. 10 screen on your face. And do not forget the wide-brimmed hat and sunglasses. They can be face-savers, too.

Patient Satisfaction

I have pointed out some of the cautions about chemabrasion and dermabrasion, but I must also tell you that patient satisfaction with these procedures runs high. More and more people are turning to them to improve facial flaws that cannot be helped by other types of cosmetic surgery. Word of mouth on these procedures has led to a major increase in the number being performed annually. Although we do not have exact statistics for the second half of this decade, we do know that, during the first half of the eighties, over 50,000 such procedures were being performed each year and that the number continues to grow. Between 1981 and 1984, the number of chemical peels done in this country increased by 67 percent; the number of dermabrasions by 38 percent. Furthermore, as the number of physicians trained in these procedures increases, I believe an ever-growing number of people will undergo them.

Two years ago I took early retirement from my office job with AT&T, a job I had held for longer than I care to remember. I was looking forward to my leisure, to all the idle hours I had ahead of me for the first time in my life. My husband had retired the previous year and we planned to take short and long trips, since traveling was our hobby.

Fate had different plans. My husband died suddenly, my social contacts dwindled, and I felt isolated and alone. I decided to try and get a new job. But I became aware of how my appearance had changed. I stared at myself in the mirror and noted with horror how old I looked. I had never paid much attention to what I had seen as "a few little wrinkles." Now they seemed not so few and not so little.

I realized that people in my former office probably didn't notice how much older I looked as each year went by. I had joined AT&T when I was twenty-five; now I was fifty-five. I thought I looked much more than that. And I knew that prospective employers might consider me too old for any opening they had — after all, who wants a new employee who is going to take Social Security in a few years?

Anyway, I had heard, over the years, about entertainers and women in famous positions who had their face lifted and defied nature by doing so. I went to see a highly recommended plastic surgeon who, after examining me and talking to me said that what would help me most would be an abrasion of the superficial layers of my facial skin to make my face smoother and take away some of the wrinkles. He said it would even reduce the ancient and forgotten acne scars that I still had from my teens.

Suffice it to say, I went ahead with it. There were a few unpleasant days after I got home. But now I can look in the mirror without getting depressed, and let me tell you, that's worth a lot. I must say my confidence is renewed and I even got a part-time job with a manufacturing company in my town. That operation made me feel that I'm getting a second start in life. While I have no romantic ambitions, at least at work I'm treated like one of the gang and not like somebody's rocking-chair grandmother.

I haven't had a minute's regret. In fact, I believe I traded well: a hundred little wrinkles and pits lost, for a gain of ten years.

"A beautiful face is the most beautiful of all sights."
— JEAN DE LA BRUYÈRE, *Les Caractères*

The Forehead and Brow Lift | 10

MY MOTHER IS EIGHTY-ONE *and she does push-ups. I'm fifty-eight and a grandmother and I'm going to live to be ninety-five. I just know it. I've had six children and never had any pain to speak of. I've always been very positive. I always have a good time and I'm certain that there are still plenty of good times ahead of me.*

I used to be a singer. Then I did a radio talk show for a while in Ohio. Now I'm in commercial real estate. I've had many different careers and I loved them all. I always knew when it was time to move on, though, because I think there's lots of opportunity out there and I don't want to miss out on any of it. Why should anyone do only one thing all their life? Why not four or five careers?

I had had eyelid surgery some years ago, when I was only forty-two; and I had a facelift at forty-six. Then my eyebrows began to droop a year or two ago, and I developed those unattractive forehead creases. Some people, if they live to be a hundred, don't develop those problems, but I did and I wanted to see if I could undo the ravages of time. Plastic surgery had helped me before, and I had faith that it could help me again. It did.

I had a second facelift, and with it a brow lift, which was the more important part in my case, because the top third of my face was in trouble. I feel so lucky to have had it done. I looked less than beautiful for a week or two, but that was more the facelift than the brow lift. But

I was able to laugh about it. What's a couple of weeks out of your social life if you can end up looking like I do at fifty-eight? I think life is marvelous. It's been perfect up to now and I know it's going to be even better.

My advice is not to wait too long if you have a problem that can be helped by plastic surgery. Don't wait 'til you're going on sixty. Do it at forty, and you may not stop the clock, but you sure can slow it down.

In previous chapters on facelifts and eyelid surgery, I gave you some idea of what you can expect from those procedures: tightening of the jawline and neck, removal of a double chin you've come to hate, the lifting of sagging cheeks, and elimination of the bags and pouches around your eyes. But, with time, gravity, the sun (perhaps heredity, too) all working against us, even our eyebrows and forehead have a tendency to show their age by drooping and seeming to descend lower on the face. Sometimes the brows appear to be moving closer to the eyelashes. Long horizontal creases traverse the length of the forehead. Deep frown lines between the eyes create a perpetual look of thoughtfulness, even anger . . . or the skin across the very top of the nose seems to bunch up. If you have lived long enough, there might also be a deep crease across the indentation at the top of your nose.

Fortunately there are newly evolved techniques that can halt, alter, or remove such disfiguring facial developments. The procedure is known as a *forehead and brow lift*, and it is currently being performed on approximately 10 to 15 percent of patients who undergo eyelid or facelift surgery. Actually, this procedure delivers a two-pronged benefit package: the brow lift elevates the brows, including the skin and muscles around the eyes, to retard the drooping of the brows themselves; and the forehead lift eliminates some of those forehead creases and frown lines that can be so disfiguring. The two parts of the procedure are usually done as an entity; or in conjunction with a facelift, eyelid surgery, or both.

As recently as a decade ago, attempts to raise the brows and forehead surgically were only temporarily effective and only moderately successful, if at all. But, because plastic surgery is such a rapidly progressing science, today the results from this type of cosmetic surgery are usually good *and* long-lasting.

The deep frown lines between the eyes which some people develop can make them appear angry or in deep thought, even when they are feeling very happy and carefree. A fifty-four-year-old woman who worked at Bloomingdale's in New York City (in the cosmetic department, no less!) suffered this problem. In our initial interview, she said, "I've been with the store for more than fifteen years and I have lots of friends among my coworkers. Of course, many of them are younger than I am. I truly love my work and usually feel very good when I'm there. But my friends pass my counter and say, 'Don't be so angry! Life isn't all *that* bad!' or 'Smile! The world isn't coming to an end!' These comments floor me because I'm a very upbeat person, life has been good to me, and I'm in great physical shape — unless you call my frown lines a physical breakdown. The weird thing is that those comments are made to me at times when I'm really in a very good mood. I came to see you because I thought maybe a facelift would help me."

She *was* helped by a facelift; it was relatively easy for me to predict the results since she still had good skin and a nice jawline. The facelift was combined with a forehead and brow lift, but it was the second procedure that was more instrumental in helping her regain her pleasant, youthful look. Her chronic worried face was replaced by that of a bright-looking, much younger person.

Some people, almost always women who have had one or two blepharoplasties to rid themselves of excess folds of the upper eyelids, find that their brows have dropped so much that *they* need to be lifted. Any further removal of skin from the upper eyelids would result in dropping the brows even lower and actually decreasing the distance between the upper eyelid and the eyebrow. In such cases, a brow lift can be a godsend.

This procedure involving the eyebrows and forehead is not for everyone. You may never need it, because heredity is often a major determining factor and if it's not a family trait, you may experience some degree of this cosmetic problem but not severe enough to warrant surgery. Then, there is the fact that the procedure is more complicated than some of the other facial operations described in this book, and many people choose to forgo it when their surgeon tells them what's involved.

The Technique

A description of this operation is not for the squeamish; it involves an incision across the top of the head, through the skin of the scalp, and literally a peeling down of the scalp and forehead.

I hesitate to use this analogy, but it is the best graphic description there is: peeling down the forehead is like peeling the skin from an orange, except that the surgeon keeps the peeled portion in one piece. The technique has also been referred to as the "Indian method," because it is akin to the way the Indians used to take a scalp.

Actually, there is a well-defined plane or tissue space between the skin and the soft tissue of the scalp (which includes the forehead) and the bone of the skull. This natural plane serves as an excellent guide to the surgeon and facilitates the peel. There is almost no loss of blood.

When the forehead is peeled down, the surgeon must take great care to protect the nerves that provide sensation to the forehead and scalp, as well as to the important nerve branches that help elevate the brows and squeeze closed the eyes. These muscles, which provide expression to the forehead ("His forehead wrinkled and rose in disbelief" or "Her raised eyebrows signified her surprise"), are closely attached to the skin and are separated from the bone along with the skin during the peeling process. Portions of these muscles may even be deliberately severed from the skin and permanently cut away in order to preclude further wrinkling in that region of the face.

The major muscle involved in forehead wrinkling is a large, flat, and very thin muscle that covers the entire forehead. It is aptly named the *frontalis,* since it occupies the entire front of the skull. It is the intimate relationship and interaction between the frontalis and the skin that actually creates the horizontal wrinkles across the forehead.

The deeper frown lines, especially the vertical ones, are influenced by smaller muscles that are attached to the skin in the region between the eyebrows. These small muscles are known as the *corrugator* (which literally means "the wrinkler," as in *corrugated boxes*) and the *procerus* (from the Latin, meaning "long"). They work in synergistic harmony to make us frown in order to indicate displeasure or intense thoughtfulness — sometimes even when we don't want to project those looks. Unlike other muscles, the corrugator and procerus are not essential to the functioning of the human body; we could certainly live perfectly well if they were weakened or gone completely.

After the surgeon has completed the dissection of the muscles, the forehead and scalp flap are moved back in position and put on slight tension in an upward direction. Excessive skin is removed, and the whole incision is sutured or stapled together. At this point in the operation, the surgeon must exercise great care not to stretch the skin too much; excessive tension is thought to interfere with blood supply, which can lead to loss of some of the hair follicles and, subsequently, to patches of baldness along the incision line. Sometimes these small patches of baldness occur despite all efforts to prevent them. In some people who have very high hairlines, receding hair, or areas of baldness, the incision is placed just along the edge of the hairline at the top of the forehead. Such an incision usually heals very well and is not as visible as you might imagine.

If a forehead lift is carried out at the same time as a facelift, the facelift incision that ordinarily ends in the hair-bearing scalp of the temple is simply extended up and over the top of the head, where it joins up with the facelift incision from the opposite side.

Preoperative Information

If you have a forehead and brow lift and it's combined with a facelift or a blepharoplasty, the amount of time you'll spend in the hospital or clinic is the same as if you only had the one procedure. Whichever type of anesthesia, local or general, that you and your doctor agree on for the first procedure will also be used for the second part of the operation. If you have a complete facial reconstruction — facelift, eyelids and forehead and brow — you'll probably want to have it done in a hospital and spend two or three days there. All this depends on how much work is going to be done, on your doctor's customary practice and preference, and on the ambulatory facilities available in your area for cosmetic surgery. I'd suggest that you go along with your surgeon's recommendations in matters involving anesthesia, in-hospital vs. outpatient decisions, and the advisability, in your particular case, of combining two or more procedures in a single surgical session.

BEFORE THE SURGERY

Photographs — Preoperative medical photographs are necessary so that your surgeon can study your face in detail as he plans the procedure. You won't want to put these pictures in a scrapbook — they are not meant to flatter you. But they are as essential to your surgeon as X rays are to a chest surgeon. Your doctor will either take these photographs himself or recommend a medical photographer.

Medication — To promote blood clotting, I prescribe for my patients one tablet of Vitamin K to be taken each of the three days prior to surgery, the last pill taken the day before the operation. This prescription drug is not to be taken by people with varicose veins, phlebitis, or coronary disease.

I also tell my patients to take 1,000 mg. of Vitamin C each day for at least two weeks prior to surgery. This vitamin promotes healing.

Avoiding aspirin or any aspirin-containing compound is extremely important, because it has been well established that aspirin slows down blood coagulation. There is going to be a normal amount of bleeding of the small blood vessels during surgery, and taking aspirin can increase this bleeding. Drugs that contain aspirin or aspirin compounds include Alka-Seltzer, Anacin, Bufferin, Coricidin, Darvon Compound, Dristan, Excedrin, Fiorinal, Midol, and Percodan. Anacin-3 and

Tylenol do not contain aspirin and may be taken. If you take any of the ibuprofen medications, it is probably a good idea to discontinue them forty-eight hours before surgery, unless they are badly needed for arthritis or other pain.

Smoking

You should not smoke for two weeks prior to surgery. Smoking has long been suspected as a major cause of delayed and improper wound healing. In a study of over two thousand patients, we learned that cigarette smoking was the major cause of serious wound-healing complications. If you smoke and inhale, you are at least twelve times more likely than nonsmokers to suffer poor healing of your incisions.

Paying your bill

As with all cosmetic surgery, you will probably be asked to pay your surgeon's fee in advance of the operation. If you have a general anesthetic, there will be an anesthesiologist's bill — which is usually payable before leaving the hospital or within a week of discharge.

AFTER THE SURGERY

Pain

Pain is unusual, although a small amount of pain can be experienced as a result of nerve irritation. This is temporary. In some people it lasts no more than a few hours; in others, perhaps a day or two.

Bandages

After the operation, your head will be bandaged to exert a moderate amount of compression on the skin in order to minimize the possibility of hemorrhage.

If the procedure is done in conjunction

	with a facelift, the same bandage wraps around the chin, jaws, and scalp. The bandage is removed in forty-eight hours and is not replaced.
Stitches	Stitches and staples are removed in stages — from about the sixth to twelfth days after surgery.
Bruising and swelling	In a multiple procedure, there will be a small amount of bruising and swelling but not much more than you would be likely to experience if you were to have either a facelift or eyelid surgery performed *without* work on the forehead. If work is done only on the forehead and brow, bruising will be minimal.
Makeup and shampoos	After a forehead and brow lift, makeup can be worn almost immediately after the bandage is removed. Your hair can be shampooed a week after surgery.

Possible Complications

While this should not be considered a true complication, over-elevation of the hairline can occur if the skin is stretched too much before the excess is cut away. As I mentioned previously, such overstretching can also interfere with blood supply and possibly cause some loss of hair.

One possible complication is that nerves in the forehead, although carefully protected during the surgery, must often be manipulated, and thus temporarily desensitized after the operation. This makes the area feel numb, but the feeling almost always returns unless a nerve is cut, in which case some numbness in a portion of the scalp or forehead could be permanent.

Loss of motion in the forehead region, particularly the ability to elevate the eyebrow, can happen if that branch of the facial nerve which provides motion stimuli to the brow muscle is injured. This problem is rare; when it does happen, one effective treatment calls for purposefully paralyzing the opposite brow so that the facial expression is symmetrical. I know of at least one patient in the Midwest who was delighted with the loss of motion in her brow and forehead. All of her wrinkles disappeared and she wound up with a completely smooth, if immobile, brow and forehead. It's not something we aim for, and not everyone would like that included in their surgical result — but that woman was overjoyed by it.

If the flat frontalis muscle is removed from the central area of the forehead, a slight depression can be noticed in that place. This contour depression is minimal and of little practical consequence. It is, many people think, a reasonable trade-off for getting rid of severe wrinkling.

It is not unusual for a patient to have a somewhat surprised look on his or her face for several days after surgery. Despite what you may have heard to the contrary, this is only temporary.

Alternatives to the Forehead and Brow Lift

Because of the mental image that this procedure evokes, patients for whom a forehead and brow lift is advisable often ask if there are alternative solutions. The only other treatments that can help eliminate or soften forehead wrinkles and frown lines are collagen or silicone injections. (Such injection procedures are discussed in the next chapter.) However, for deep lines, creases, and wrinkles, these techniques are no match for a surgical forehead and brow lift.

While fine lines and wrinkles, especially the very small ones that look like they have been etched in, can be improved significantly by deep chemical peeling, and to a lesser extent by dermabrasion (see Chapter 9), neither of these techniques will eliminate deep frown lines or raise a dropped eyebrow.

"Magic" creams and lotions cannot remove wrinkles and creases — despite the claims made in the advertising and publicity campaigns for such products. As one commedienne remarked when she heard about a wrinkle-remover product made with turtle oil, "I never saw a good-looking turtle; or, for that matter, one without wrinkles."

Looking over the Results

The results of a forehead and brow lift can be classified as "good" to "excellent." This procedure is definitely worthwhile for people with deep frown lines, horizontal forehead creases and furrows, or dropped eyebrows. What the operation does is give the fully recovered patient a softer, more youthful appearance around the brows and forehead, restore a slipped eyebrow to its former, more elevated position, and alleviate or eliminate frown lines. There is an extra dividend that can be expected from this operation. As a result of the elevated brows, more of the upper lid shows, and the bony contour of the eye's orbit becomes more distinct. This always makes the person appear more youthful and alert.

If you have some of the facial characteristics that are indications for a forehead and brow lift, and if you would like to have an idea of what this type of surgery could do for you, try this demonstration: Look in the mirror and put the heels of your hands on your forehead, just above the eyebrows. Then, slide your forehead skin upwards. Take note of the new position of your eyebrows and what it does for the youthfulness of your face. This demonstration will give you a general idea of what you can expect from the surgery.

How long the results of a forehead and brow lift will last depends on the individual's tendency to show age, on heredity, the condition of the skin, and the presence or absence of other physical ailments or diseases. In a healthy, generally upbeat person who has managed to carry his or her youthfulness well beyond the beginning of middle age, the prognosis for long-range success is excellent.

I was a very successful model, although I stopped modeling years ago and went into daytime soaps. Being an actress and a model makes you very aware of your looks and of the aging process. The roles you're offered are directly connected to your looks. The writer, the director, the casting department, the producer — everyone thinks first of how an actress <u>looks</u> and then how well she acts. But that's the business, and I'm not saying it's the wrong way to cast a part; it's just a fact of life.

I had had two facelifts, both very successful, and at the time of my second surgery, I was already well into my fifties and figured it was my last cosmetic operation in <u>this</u> life. As I approached my sixties, I

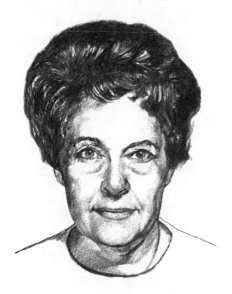 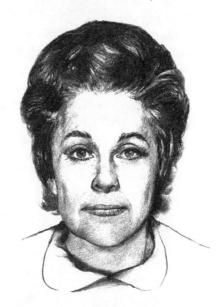

This patient had a facelift and a forehead and brow lift. With age, her brows had fallen, but surgery restored them to a more elevated and natural position, promoting a more youthful appearance.

found that no amount of makeup could conceal the ridges developing in my forehead, or the grooves about the place where my eyeglasses fit on my face. I thought maybe I had taken to frowning, unknowingly, while wearing reading glasses, so I switched to contact lenses.

The problem didn't get better, and I went back to the surgeon who had done my second facelift. People in my profession talk a lot about plastic surgery, the men as well as the women, but I had never heard of a forehead lift. And when the doctor suggested I was a good candidate for a combination eyelid operation and forehead lift, I was, frankly, stunned. I told him I'd think about it.

Well, maybe I've always been a little avant-garde, in my clothes and my hairstyles and my whole life-style, in fact. I trusted my doctor, and I figured if I didn't have it done I'd soon be wearing a couple of inches of pancake makeup to hide those furrows. So I signed on.

Looking at me now, it's probably difficult to imagine what I looked like before. But if you saw the medical "before" pictures, you wouldn't believe it's the same person. The puffs are gone because of the eyelid surgery, and I've gotten rid of most of those darn <u>wrinkles</u> in my forehead. The whole top half of my face seems to give me a younger look. At least, I think so. Everyone at work thinks I had a facelift because the top part of my face is so smooth, almost no wrinkles.

And it wasn't at all a bad experience. I was up and around a mere twenty-four hours after surgery, and comfortable about going out in public in about two weeks. They told me that many people go through a slight depression after cosmetic surgery. Not me. I'm elated. Who knows what they'll come up with next!

"You can tell a woman's beauty by reading between the lines."
— CECIL BEATON, QUOTED IN HUGO VICKERS,
Cecil Beaton: A Biography

Silicone and Collagen Treatments   11

I COME FROM A YOUTHFUL FAMILY. *Everyone in my family always looked much younger than they actually were. My grandmother, who died at ninety-one, could have passed for a woman a dozen years younger. My mother, at fifty-eight, had fine, clear skin, without any wrinkles at all. Her blue eyes were clear, no bags or puffs underneath. Her brown hair hadn't a gray one in her whole head. She works for the State Department, writing press releases, and when I visit her at her office, people sometimes ask if we're sisters.*

Unfortunately, bad teeth also run in my family and, though fifty-eight is very young for such a thing, she had to have her lower teeth taken out and replaced with a denture. You couldn't tell she wore a denture because it was well concealed by her lower lip. But a strange thing happened. Within a year, she developed wrinkles on her lower jaw, around the jawline. It was really weird: the rest of her face was so young looking and just that small part of her face with wrinkles.

It bothered Mom, and her older sister (who, by the time Mom's wrinkles developed, looked like her younger sister) told her to see a plastic surgeon about the possibility of a facelift, which my mother did. He didn't think a facelift was the answer to her problem, but he suggested she have collagen injections, to be given in two sessions, two weeks apart. After the first session, she developed a slight lumpiness, very slight, but the doctor told her it would go away, which it did. He postponed the second session until three weeks after the first.

It's now about eight months since she had the injections and she is one hundred percent glad that she had it done. She has a good complexion, very fine skin, and still you can't see any marks where it was done — at least I can't see any. Since the rest of her face has remained very young and unwrinkled, this correction on the jawline actually turned back the clock for her. She's pleased as punch with the results. She says my aunt deserves a medal for suggesting my mother go to a plastic surgeon.

As we grow older, the skin begins to dry out and the lines and creases in the face grow more prominent. Our bones, fat, and muscles gradually shrink while the aging skin is inclined to stretch so that it no longer fits the underlying tissues as tightly as it did when we were young. Add to that the downward pull of gravity and the effects of exposure to the sun, and you can see that the skin truly takes a beating over time.

I have told you about a number of surgical procedures that can be helpful in tightening a sagging skin, erasing or diminishing wrinkles and lines, and in abrading surface scars and certain pigmentation changes. But there are a number of "contour" problems — those involving depressions or hollow areas of the face — that are not always amenable to surgery, peeling, or abrasion. Fortunately, medical and scientific advances in recent years have added additional procedures to our storehouse of medical techniques so that we can, nowadays, often improve these conditions or even eliminate some of them. In this chapter, I will tell you about the current state of the art in using silicone and collagen to correct certain anatomical problems when surgery, peeling, or abrasion is not indicated.

For centuries, a safe "filler" substance had been sought, one that could be implanted in the body by injecting it through the skin, without giving rise to undesirable reactions such as inflammation, infection, "migrating" (or dislocation), or total rejection. Ideally, such a substance would not deteriorate with time, would not encourage bacterial growth, and would, of course, be noncarcinogenic. This is a large order for any injected substance to fill.

Through the years, many different substances — both biological and synthetic — were tried. In this search for the ideal injectable material, a number of high-viscosity liquids of animal and vegetable origin were employed as tissue substitutes, most of them unsatisfactory because of the adverse reactions they set off in the body.

The best-known and most widely used of these materials was liquid paraffin. As early as the turn of this century, a Czechoslovakian doctor named Robert Gersuny reported that he had avoided surgery on a patient by using this substance as a contour filler. (At that time, the round face was in vogue, considered to be a sign of youth and health. Had today's gaunt-looking American model appeared on the scene, she would have been suspected of having tuberculosis.) A number of prominent people, eager to rid themselves of hollows and wrinkles, had themselves injected with liquid paraffin, often by nonphysicians, since surgical training was not required for the administration of this procedure.

Reports, however, very soon told of unfortunate consequences from using liquid paraffin: the formation of lumps and bumps (benign *paraffin granulomas*), repeated bouts of swelling and redness in the injected areas, and sometimes pain. Often the treatment was worse than the problem for which the patient had sought help. As the reports increased, responsible physicians abandoned the use of paraffin, although even today there are still some nonlicensed practitioners, and even some doctors in Hong Kong, Singapore, Southeast Asia, and Taiwan, who use it, either ignorant or indifferent to the problems it creates. I must advise you to steer clear of anyone who suggests the use of paraffin as material to be injected in your face, or anywhere else in your body, for that matter.

One well-known case of a person whose face was ravaged by paraffin injections was the Duchess of Marlborough, who in her youth was a reigning beauty of London society. To achieve a fuller face, she had multiple injections of liquid paraffin, and the results were disastrous. Both her great beauty and her social life were destroyed. She died a recluse at her country estate, having for years been afraid to show her face in public.

After the failure of paraffin liquid, a number of other substances enjoyed temporary vogue. These materials included lanolin and various vegetable oils, but they, too, were poorly tolerated by human tissues and were discarded as showing no promise for cosmetic purposes.

Silicone Fluid

In the mid-1950s, rumors began to reach the medical profession of a new liquid mixture that was being used in Europe and the Orient to fill in wrinkles and skin depressions on the face, as well as to augment small breasts.

At first, it was practically impossible to obtain scientific data about this mysterious substance, but, after long and painstaking investigation, it was finally identified by the medical profession as *liquid* silicone. We already knew of *solid* silicone, a man-made plastic compound that causes minimal reaction in the body, has the ability to remain in place during a recipient's lifetime, and is generally well tolerated. Today, solid silicone is in wide use for implants under the skin, on the chin, nose, ears, and other locations. It is used as bone and cartilage substitutes in surgical procedures requiring implants that include heart valves, artificial joints, pacemakers, breast prostheses, artificial blood vessels, and so on.

It is not uncommon for people to confuse silicone (spelled with an *e*) with *silicon*. While silicone is man-made, silicon is found everywhere in nature. It is best known as a component of ordinary sand, from which glass is made. Silicone is manufactured by the Dow Corning Corporation and is used for medical purposes in every known physical form, ranging from liquid to a gel to a solid substance.

The silicone fluid that was being used in the 1950s was diluted with an additive to cause an inflammatory reaction to the tissues on the theory that this would make the results more permanent. A Japanese mixture, one in which an oil was added to the pure silicone fluid, was in wide use in Asia. Named after a Japanese doctor, it was called the *Sakurai formula*.

Today, the use of silicone as a solid is not controversial. However, while it is well tolerated by the body, it does have one principal enemy: infection. Sometimes it becomes necessary to remove the implant when infection occurs around it; but then, no implant material has yet been devised that is 100 percent nonreactive. An inflammatory response is the body's attempt to wall off foreign material, and this results in the formation of scar tissue around the invader. The principal component of this scar tissue is collagen, a substance which, in itself, is today being used as an injectable tissue filler. (In the second part of this chapter I will discuss collagen.)

In many different studies and animal experiments conducted in universities and laboratories, silicone fluid was found to offer promise as a soft tissue filler, and during the sixties it was in wide use as an injectable for the purpose of increasing breast size. It has been said that, at one point in the 1960s, one out of five showgirls in Las Vegas had probably received silicone injections into her breasts. As a matter of fact, its use was so widespread that the state of Nevada passed a law making it illegal to inject silicone for this purpose.

Injection of the large volume of silicone required to increase breast size caused major tissue response, in which breasts became hard, lumpy, painful, and swollen. After months, sometimes years, injected breasts often became rock-hard and full of lumps, much like a sack filled with different-sized rocks. In addition, the skin assumed the texture and appearance of an orange peel. (Referred to medically as "peau d'orange," this condition is created when the skin swells with fluid as the tiny lymph ducts in the breast become obstructed by the silicone.)

Today, there is complete agreement among physicians that liquid silicone, injected for the purpose of breast augmentation, is unsuitable. However, this substance has proven effective and safe when treating certain diseases that cause atrophy of the face, particularly when such atrophy occurs on only one side. For other applications of this material, disagreement among the experts continues. Some are unequivocally enthusiastic about it; others disapprove. Those who are in favor of liquid silicone injections maintain that success or failure does not depend on the substance itself, but on the way it is used.

Such injections have, in point of fact, proven to be a godsend for some people afflicted with facial problems for which surgery is not helpful, such as facial atrophy (particularly when it is one-sided) and congenital defects. If you are an older person and the fat pads in your cheeks have shrunk or become absorbed into the body, creating depressions just beneath the cheekbones, liquid silicone injections could be something a plastic surgeon or dermatologist might recommend to you.

The principal disadvantage of silicone injection treatment is that the material cannot be removed once it has been put in place, except by surgery. It is permanently there, within the tissues.

Since the FDA has classified liquid silicone as a drug, not as an injectable prosthesis, Dow Corning has not yet produced or marketed silicone fluid that can be injected for medical purposes. As of this writing, a carefully selected research team of doctors appointed by the American Society of Plastic and Reconstructive Surgeons is studying the use of silicone under clinical conditions. They are examining the advisability of using liquid silicone injections to solve some of the serious medical problems of the face I mentioned above, which cannot be treated successfully by other means. However, *wrinkles of the skin do not qualify as serious enough to be part of this study.*

This type of research effort is always necessary before any new drug can be released for general medical use. The Federal Food and Drug Administration requires exhaustive research, both in the laboratory and in human patients, to prove that a drug is safe and effective and has no effect on the growth and development of a fetus. Currently, there are also studies underway by independent researchers and by the Dow Corning Corporation, to learn more about liquid silicone.

I doubt that the use of silicone fluid for the treatment of wrinkles will ever be officially approved, even though it is effective for this purpose. The substance has had too much negative publicity regarding its misuse in breasts. One would think that this publicity would deter people from seeking *any* treatment employing a silicone product. Of course, the complications resulting from the massive doses injected into the breasts do not apply to the treatment of minor facial defects such as wrinkles, which require comparatively minuscule quantities.

Even though liquid silicone has not been approved by the FDA as an injectable for medical purposes, and despite the fact that the Dow Corning Corporation is not marketing such a product for medical use, many doctors, both here and abroad, are using silicone to plump out wrinkles for their patients. The fact that a drug is not FDA-approved does not mean it's illegal to use it. However, doctors who do use liquid silicone recognize that they are assuming responsibility for the treatment and, should a complication occur, they have no protection from a medical/legal point of view. Silicone has many commercial uses that have no relationship to medicine or cosmetic surgery, and it is fairly easy to obtain the industrial-grade fluid on the open market, purify it by filtering and sterilizing, and then use it for injection. The actual process of injecting this substance is very simple, which is what makes it so appealing to physicians worldwide. Technically, it is not illegal to inject liquid silicone, so there are some reputable and well-accredited physicians in this country who do use it. Although no hard data are available, I think it is safe to say that millions of people in the U.S., Europe, and Asia have received silicone injections for the treatment of wrinkles and minor facial defects. Unfortunately, a wholly unbiased analysis of the results of its use for such purposes has been difficult to come by. Accurate reporting on its long-term success or failure as a substance to "fill" wrinkles is nonexistent.

The Silicone Injection Procedure

Silicone injection is a relatively simple procedure which does not require hospitalization. In most patients no premedication is required. A local anesthesia is not given, either, since injection into the tissues would distort the feature or the part of the face that's being worked on. After cleansing the face with an antiseptic solution, a limited number of droplets (anywhere from ten to twenty) are injected beneath the skin. Each drop is injected separately and spaced along each wrinkle or depression being treated. The procedure is done with a fine needle, very slowly, and the area is then gently massaged by the surgeon or nurse to achieve an even distribution of the silicone. The small drops are soon locked in place by the surrounding fibrous tissues.

Pain, even discomfort, is rare after the procedure. Some swelling or discoloration may occur, but this is short-lived, lasting a day or two at the most.

While the effects of this procedure are long-lasting, wrinkles continue to develop and, over a period of time, a repetition of the process may be necessary.

What I have described pertains only to the injection of minute amounts of silicone for the purpose of correcting small wrinkles. When larger volumes are used to correct facial atrophy or other significant contour deformities of the face, the injection technique differs considerably. Treating such problems calls for the injection of several milliliters into the subcutaneous layer beneath the skin. The injections are not given all at once; treatment sessions are spaced over a period of many weeks. As the doctor injects these larger volumes, he moves his needle constantly in order to distribute the silicone fluid evenly beneath the skin, thus minimizing the chance of "pooling," which could eventually lead to the formation of lumps. After each treatment, the injected area is vigorously massaged by a vibrating machine to further ensure even distribution of the fluid throughout the tissues.

The Results

Most patients receiving liquid silicone injections are happy with the results. Jillian, a California woman who came to see me about a facelift, had previously had silicone injections by a West Coast physician, and the procedure had succeeded in filling out some deep frown lines she had between her eyes. "I cannot even point to the precise spot where the injections were made," she told me, "although, of course, I know the area that was worked on. After a few weeks, I almost forgot that the treatment had taken place. I only know that the furrow bothered me terribly or I wouldn't have gone to a doctor."

Jillian was a healthy, athletic woman in her early fifties, a homemaker for her four children and her husband, a golf pro. She was an avid tennis player who was on the courts almost every day, and she felt that squinting in the sun for hours at a time, over a period of many years, had contributed to her former problem. She said that since her injection therapy she wore sunglasses outdoors whenever possible, or used a sun-block cream. In the thirty years since Jillian had moved to the West Coast from New York, she had seen a lot of sun and surf, and her skin was quite dried out and prematurely wrinkled. She didn't get a facelift — she had no jowls and her skin had not sagged — but she did have a chemical peel, with results that she found very pleasing, although that procedure was more uncomfortable and the recovery period much longer than she had experienced with the silicone injections.

Perhaps the largest experience in the world with silicone injections used for the treatment of wrinkles has been gained in New York City, where several prominent and well-regarded dermatologists champion this technique. I have personally seen hundreds of patients who have had silicone injections for this purpose and well over a hundred who have had major volumes of silicone injected for the treatment of major facial deformities. In this large group of patients, I have seen surprisingly few complications; in fact, fewer than I would have anticipated. While I certainly do not mean this to be an endorsement of silicone injection treatments which have not been FDA-approved, I must tell you that I do believe this therapy should have a definite place in cosmetic medical practice. If the material were used only when properly indicated, and administered with caution and good technique, I would expect there to be no more complications experienced from this treatment than from surgical treatments such as dermabrasion, chemical peeling, or knife surgery.

Common Myths about Silicone Injections

I've said that silicone fluid does not travel or drift through the body after injection by proper technique. Yet the belief that it does is very common. *If* injected in small amounts by a skilled and experienced physician, the fluid stays exactly where it was injected.

Some people believe that silicone fluid will eventually cause problems in the body if you wait long enough. The evidence does not show this to be the case. As with any surgical procedure, a small percentage of people who undergo this treatment will experience complications (about 4 percent with this procedure) which are more likely to occur if the material injected was adulterated — not medically pure.

There is also the myth which says that a surgeon wishing to remove injected silicone can stick a needle in and draw off the liquid. Not true. Once injected into the tissue, it is broken up into thousands of minute globules of fluid and becomes part of a latticework of fibrous tissue that can only be removed by surgery, along with the tissue in which it's imbedded.

Another myth tells us that silicone fluid causes an allergic response in the body. To the contrary, research shows that this substance is biologically inert and, as such, cannot challenge the body's immune system or instigate an allergic response.

The worst myth of all, because it is so off-putting and there is no evidence to support it, is that silicone fluid can cause cancer. Again — it is an inert substance, and a great deal of animal experimentation has failed to link the formation of cancer cells to the presence of silicone fluid in the tissues.

Collagen: What It Is . . . What It Does

No one is comfortable with the idea of injecting a man-made plastic fluid into the body that cannot be wholly retrieved. Even though silicone fluid has proven to be successful for the treatment of many contour defects and certain wrinkles, the search for a *biological* injectable material continues. By *biological* we mean a material derived from animal, plant, or human (not man-made) that can be truly incorporated into the body tissues. Ideally, such a substance, should it incite an allergic response, would be destroyed, absorbed, or replaced by the body's natural defense mechanism.

The duty of the body's defense (or immune) mechanism is to search out and destroy foreign protein. This is known as an *immune response* or an *allergic response.* Most of the biological materials that have in the past been considered as implant materials have acted as allergens — that is, they've triggered an allergic response in the body. By contrast, many nonbiologic substances (also called *nonprotein* substances) are well tolerated by humans because they are biologically inert. Silicone, as I said previously, is one such substance.

And so, the search has gone on: find a suitable biologic injectable derived from animal tissue or plant life that will be incorporated into the body after injection without triggering allergic reactions. This sounds like a simple challenge but it is, in fact, very difficult to accomplish.

The biggest breakthrough in this search has come in the form of injectable collagen. Collagen is a substance found throughout human and animal tissue. The word itself is derived from the Greek word for glue. Collagen is the glue of all the tissues in the body — literally what holds us together. It is the protein in our skin and in our connective tissue that provides the structural support for skin, cartilage, muscles, tendons, and even bone. When a wound in our body heals, it is collagen that is produced by the tissue cells to bind the wound together, fill in the spaces, and provide tensile strength. Unfortunately, as we get older, we experience a certain amount of collagen loss in the skin, and it is this loss that causes wrinkling, sagging, and various other signs of aging. One of the reasons I speak so often in this book about the need to protect ourselves from the sun is that the collagen content in the body is decreased when the skin is damaged by solar rays, making it sag and wrinkle prematurely.

It follows naturally that great effort has been directed toward the restoration of depleted collagen. While we have been unable to produce precisely the same type of collagen that the body has lost, years of exploration and experimentation led, in the mid-seventies, to the development of a purified collagen that is a natural animal protein made from the skin of cattle. This bovine collagen is scientifically treated and purified so that its allergenic properties are almost totally removed. It is kept suspended in a solution of saline or natural salt water until used, and then it is injected through a small hypodermic needle.

Before bovine collagen was developed as an injectable, animal collagen had been used in medicine for a variety of purposes, the most common of which were heart-valve prostheses and surgical sutures. The collagen now in use for aesthetic procedures is called Zyderm Collagen and is produced by the Collagen Corporation of California. Recently, this company introduced Zyderm II, a somewhat thicker solution, and GAX, an even thicker solution. The company began amassing clinical data on their product in 1978 and research is ongoing, but the substance was officially approved by the FDA in 1981.

Before You Are Scheduled for Collagen Treatment

For the vast majority of patients, collagen, used as an injectable to eliminate wrinkles and plump out depressions of the face, seems to be relatively free of complications. However, there are rare individuals who show allergic responses to the material. These people seem to be allergic to certain proteins derived from cows.

Before suggesting collagen treatments, your physician will take a detailed medical history to determine if there's any history of severe allergies or whether you suffer from such autoimmune diseases as rheumatoid arthritis. These are contraindications for the collagen procedure.

It is also necessary to do a small skin test thirty days before a collagen treatment. This test is simple and harmless enough — much like the skin test for tuberculosis. Your doctor will inject a small amount of collagen into your arm, and you'll then be asked to watch the spot for a month to see if there's any reaction. A positive skin reaction manifests itself in a firm reddish nodule at the site of the needle puncture. Although such tests are not 100 percent reliable, they do serve to eliminate, for the most part, those people for whom collagen is definitely not indicated. However, in my experience, approximately 2 percent of patients with a negative skin test will still turn out to be allergic to collagen.

THE COLLAGEN INJECTION PROCEDURE

Injectable collagen implants act as a replacement for the collagen in the deep layers of skin that have been damaged or lost as a result of aging, disease, or a birth defect. The technique differs from the silicone injection procedure in that it's injected *into* the deep layers of the skin, whereas silicone is injected *just beneath* the skin.

Since almost 80 percent of the injected material is a saline solution, which disappears through absorption within a few days of the injection, the procedure calls for overcorrection at the time it's administered. When the thicker Zyderm II is used, it takes considerably longer for the treated area to smooth out; sometimes it remains lumpy for several weeks.

Often the technique calls for more than one treatment session. While some minor problems can be corrected or improved in a single procedure, two to six sessions are more likely. The number of treatments depends on the size of the problem. Injections are given at least two weeks apart, in the doctor's office or in an outpatient clinic. Hospitalization is not necessary and no anesthesia is required. The technique is surprisingly easy, and most physicians have their nurse or trained technician administer the injections. Except when unusually large areas are to be injected, most patients need to plan only a short interruption of their customary social and business activities.

It appears from experience with tens of thousands of people who have already had collagen injections that the material warms to body temperature, becomes stationary, and is then fixed in the tissues. It is not subject to migration. Within a matter of weeks, the injected area of skin assumes the appearance and texture of normal healthy skin. When seen under a microscope, the collagen implant appears like a latticework of collagen fibers that has been compared to the threads in a piece of fabric. In fact, the microscopic appearance is almost indistinguishable from normal collagen in the skin. In time, the recipient's own cells and blood vessels develop around the collagen network.

A new, thicker form of collagen, called Zyplast, has been developed, and more and more clinical evidence is accumulating that shows it to be effective in treating larger facial defects such as atrophy. However, as this book is being written, the final word on this form of collagen is not yet in.

Possible Complications

The allergic reactions to collagen that I am aware of are mild in nature: a lump at the site of injection, or some redness. I know of no severe reactions to collagen injections although the manufacturer of Zyderm tells us it is not to be used on people with active inflammatory skin conditions (cysts, pimples, rashes, or hives) or people suffering infections — at least until these problems have gone away. The use of Zyderm is also not recommended for infants, children, and pregnant women.

One of the small problems associated with these injections is that there is gradual absorption of the material in the body and over a period of months, the favorable effects achieved will be diminished, or even disappear, with time. Many physicians believe that the injected collagen implant is eventually absorbed completely by the body, and its cosmetic effect is lost. In general, however, patients have been quite satisfied with the results of these treatments; the physicians who administered them have been less satisfied. Many people do not seem to worry about what will happen in a year or two; if they have an immediate cosmetic problem that distresses them, and if the negative effects of the treatment are not dangerous or life-threatening, they seem willing to have the treatment and perhaps repeat it in years to come. I have had patients who, when told that the results will not be everlasting, say, "So what? If it's all absorbed in months or years, I'll come back and get some more." This is one of the principal differences between silicone and collagen. Once silicone is injected into the tissues, it is permanently in place and will not break down in the body. Continuing research may well prduce a form of collagen that remains in the tissue and is not eventually absorbed. The result would then be permanent.

The Collagen Myths

Don't believe the advertisements which promise you can replace the collagen content of the tissues by applying some product externally. Collagen is *not* absorbed through the skin. It simply cannot migrate from a cosmetic on the face, through the skin barrier, and then reinforce the collagen network in your tissues. Any such promise should be ignored.

It is equally untrue that collagen can be effective if taken by mouth — it would be completely destroyed by your digestive enzymes.

Many people also believe that collagen is effective in treating acne scars. Actually, it depends largely on the type of scar. The deep, so-called ice-pick scars do not respond to collagen. They can only be treated by surgical removal. The only type of acne scar that can be improved by collagen is the shallow crater, particularly those that have softened over the years.

Another bit of misinformation is that people who have previously had silicone injections cannot have collagen treatments. That used to be the case, but considerable experimental work with collagen has shown that it's perfectly safe for you to have both. It has been demonstrated that the two substances are well tolerated side by side.

The most persistent myth about collagen is that the results are permanent. I wish this were so — it is not. No one knows for certain, but the evidence seems to indicate that the injected collagen is absorbed sooner or later; perhaps not the entire injected volume, but certainly a large part of it. Some beneficial effects seem to remain, and booster injections six to twenty-four months after the original procedure can augment and sustain the favorable results.

Finally, we have the oft-repeated myth that collagen is a chemical miracle that is going to replace facelift surgery. This is absolutely untrue. Each procedure is designed for a specific purpose. Sagging tissues cannot be tightened by collagen. Only small wrinkles, surface scars, and other minor contour defects can be improved by the collagen procedure and the results vary greatly, person to person.

The Outlook for Collagen

Since injectable collagen was approved by the FDA only in 1981, we have had a relatively short period of time in which to evaluate the long-term effects of this substance. But results do appear to be very promising, if not permanent. Most people are not allergic to this animal protein and, with rare exception, those who undergo the procedure say they are happy with the outcome.

While collagen is no substitute for facelifts, brow lifts, eyelid plasty, peels, abrasions, and other surgical procedures, I believe we can look forward to continued progress in the use of this substance for cosmetic purposes.

Ellen, a patient in her sixties who had had a successful facelift eight months previously, felt that she would like to blur the "aging lines" around her mouth — the two perioral lines that go from the corners of the mouth downwards to the chin. Such lines are not eliminated by a facelift; although, occasionally, as the jawline is tightened, the lines become less noticeable.

After collagen injections, here is what Ellen said:

I was quite happy with my facelift; a lot <u>more</u> than "happy," in fact. I was <u>overjoyed</u> that a woman like me, already past sixty, could once again have such a firm, neat neck and jawline.

But, having become so aware of the effects of aging on my looks, the thought of possibly eliminating those down lines as well was my incentive to go through another procedure. If the facelift took ten years off my looks, the collagen treatments took off a few more. It was the right way to go. My face looks simply great.

"You can call anybody an ugly duckling but an ugly duckling."
— WILL ROGERS

Improving the Ear through Surgery | 12

*F*ROM THE TIME HE WAS *four years old, we knew that my son, Billy, had ears that stood out and seemed the wrong size for his head. We thought he would just outgrow it. He was the apple of our eye and we thought he was adorable, protruding ears and all.*

Things changed, however, when he entered school at the age of six. He was outstanding in the first grade — not for his achievements, but for his ears, as evidenced by the unpleasant nicknames bestowed on him. I don't care to repeat them but they were mean enough to make me cringe. Imagine the effect they had on Billy!

It seemed that his classmates saw none of Billy's good features. They saw only his ears. We tried to get him to laugh it off with us, but it didn't work. He insisted I let him grow his hair longer and whenever possible, he wore a cap with earflaps that covered his ears. Much to our dismay and displeasure, he even wore his winter hat or earmuffs when he was indoors.

When we saw that the effect of the schoolyard teasing was having a lasting effect on Billy, we asked his pediatrician for advice and she, without hesitating, referred us to a plastic surgeon for consultation.

We didn't have to coax Billy at all. To the contrary, he agreed immediately to an operation. It was done in July, and by the time he went back to school in September, his classmates didn't seem to remember his former nicknames. They probably found some new target for their gibes. And the surgery certainly had more than a physical effect on Billy. For one thing, no more caps. For another, he didn't come home from school every day in tears. He became more self-confident and began to participate more in group sports.

It seems to my husband and me like a short episode in our lives, and we are gradually forgetting that first year of Billy's schooling. He appears to have completely forgotten the protruding ears he was born with. From what I know now, had I to do it over again, I wouldn't waste a minute on weighing the pros and cons. That operation was, in Billy's case, an absolute necessity. If someone who had a child with protruding ears came to me for advice, I would immediately say, "Go ahead! Find a good surgeon and have the ears operated on. You won't regret it!"

Take a good look at your ear. You probably never thought about it this way, but isn't that ear a great work of art? It's a sculpture so delicate, such a superbly designed configuration of angles and folds, that even the most accomplished of artists would have a difficult time designing a functional organ more pleasing to the eye. Most people will recognize that they have pretty eyes, or a handsome nose, or a lovely mouth, or perhaps nice high cheekbones. But it does not occur to most of us to acknowledge what a superb work of art we have on either side of our head.

When I say "functional" I mean, of course, that it is more than a decorative feature of the human body. Nature gave us the external ear (*auricle*) to protect the drum and middle ear (*tympanum*) and the inner ear (*labyrinth*) from damage and to act as a funnel that feeds and filters sound from the outside.

The external ear is made of a tough, elastic cartilage covered by a thin, fibrous envelope of skin. The earlobe, however, is all soft tissue, skin, and fat — no cartilage. The ear structure differs from person to person almost as much as do fingerprints. In fact, the left and right ears of any one individual differ even from each other. Most people don't know this because they've never spent much time scrutinizing this feature. Incidentally, the look of the ears also differs race to race. Polynesians, for example, generally have large ears, while those of Africans are proportionally small. The attachment of the earlobes to the head also varies race to race.

The only people who pay much attention to their ears are those who suffer some deformity or cosmetic imperfection of one or both of them. Protruding ears — where the ears stand away from the head to a degree that is greater than normal — are the most common imperfection on this part of the body and they are found in more than 5 percent of the human race, although some cultures do not consider them to be either a flaw or a deformity. Medically speaking, protruding ears are *not* a true physical deformity, albeit they often create psychological problems.

There are, of course, numerous other ear imperfections, some genetic in origin, some caused by accidents or other traumas. I will discuss these later on in this chapter. I believe it would be correct to assume, however, that if you are reading this chapter, you are probably more interested in knowing what can be done about protruding ears — a condition that occurs with much greater frequency than all other ear deformities put together. In my practice, through the years, over 95 percent of the people who have come to see me about ear problems of their own or their children have come for that reason. Four out of five concern children.

One would think protruding ears to be a lesser cosmetic flaw, one that could easily be disregarded. Such is not the case for the multitude of youngsters who, at an early age, begin to suffer the caustic comments of play- and classmates. The fact that protruding ears on a small boy's head (most girls with this problem manage to grow their hair so that it covers the ears) are noticeable in the first school years is most unfortunate because this is a time in life when one's peers can be bluntly outspoken, often unkind by adult standards. Children with protruding ears are tagged with a variety of cruel nicknames. "Dumbo" may be an amusing name for an elephant in a Walt Disney cartoon, but a small child with such a nickname invariably suffers pain, even if he displays an outward buffoonery — probably a disguise to cover his inward agony. Distasteful jokes are commonplace. "Why don't you flap your ears and fly?" an uninhibited youngster might shout to his playmate. Children can be very mean in expressing their evaluation of the physical traits of their comrades. Withholding the truth to avoid hurting someone's feelings is a learned skill. Continued teasing and ridicule can have a lasting effect on a child's self esteem, leaving lifelong battle scars, and it is for this reason that parents will bring their youngsters to a plastic surgeon for consultation. As one six-year-old said to me, "The other kids all poke fun at me. I don't want to be poked."

Sometimes, parents come in with their children only after they have tried other home-made remedies without success, such as taping back the child's ears or having him sleep for months with a nightcap or a kerchief tied around the head. These devices obviously have no effect. Corrective surgery is the only way to bring about a physical change as well as psychological relief from the child's keenly felt anguish.

Most of the patients who visit surgeons for help with their protruding ears are young, although not all of them are small children. People in middle age and older are rarely concerned with this problem, having learned to live with their ears.

Correction of protruding ears by an operation called *otoplasty* saves the youthful patient from years of further humiliation. If surgery is postponed beyond childhood, it can still be carried out at almost any age. Because the ears are almost fully grown long before the rest of the body (by the age of five), they may sometimes look disproportionately big on a child and even a slight variation from the norm in the way they protrude can make them appear abnormal. Surgery does not interfere with further growth of the ears, so it is not unusual to perform this type of operation when a child is anywhere from four to six, preferably before entrance into school.

BEFORE THE SURGERY

Photographs — Very likely, your surgeon (or your child's) will want to have medical photographs taken before surgery. If the surgeon doesn't take them himself, he will probably recommend a special medical photographer. The pictures will be full-face, side view, and probably rear view. Your surgeon will take these photos to the operating room for reference, if necessary.

Medication	For my adult patients, I prescribe three tablets of Vitamin K, to be taken every morning for three days prior to the operation, with the last pill taken the day before surgery. This vitamin facilitates blood clotting. You need a prescription for it, and it's not to be taken by anyone with varicose veins or a history of coronary disease or phlebitis. For adult patients, 1,000 mg. of Vitamin C each day for at least two weeks prior to surgery, is helpful in promoting healing. I do not prescribe either of these vitamins for children because of the impending surgery. Neither children nor adults should take aspirin or any aspirin-containing compound for two weeks before surgery and for a week after it. Among the over-the-counter drugs to be avoided are Alka-Seltzer, Anacin, Bufferin, Coricidin, Darvon Compound, Dristan, Excedrin, Fiorinal, Midol, and Percodan. Anacin-3 and Tylenol do not contain aspirin. Anyone taking an ibuprofen medication should probably discontinue it for forty-eight hours prior to surgery, unless it's needed for arthritis or other pain. The reason aspirin and other medications that contain aspirin are to be avoided is that they slow down blood coagulation by interfering with the ability of the platelets in the blood to adhere to each other and form a blood clot. Good healing depends on blood coagulating properly.
Where the operation is performed	This procedure can be performed either on an ambulatory, outpatient basis, or in a hospital. If you are a parent whose child

is the patient, you will need to decide whether your child might be frightened by a hospital stay. Children today see so much television involving hospital settings and operating rooms that they are a good deal more blasé about these environments than their parents or grandparents.

If the operation is performed in a hospital, a one-day stay is all that's required. If your insurance doesn't cover aesthetic surgery, the cost of hospitalization is a factor you may want to consider in deciding whether the procedure should be done in-hospital or on an outpatient basis.

About the Anesthesia

Otoplasty can be performed under local anesthesia even in children, if they are cooperative. However, if a youngster is likely to feel terrified, general anesthesia can be used. Where adults are concerned, most surgeons will recommend a local anesthesia unless a patient doesn't want to be even slightly aware of being in an operating room. Even under a local, however, you (or your child) will be mostly "out of it," having been adequately sedated in advance.

If you are thinking of this operation for a child, the prime consideration should, obviously, be the well-being of the child. It has been my experience that the great majority of children do a good job of coping with their apprehensions, and they soon forget all about the operation, no matter where it was performed. (In fact, children very quickly forget what their ears looked like *before* the surgery.) I have never known a child to be psychologically scarred by the experience of this procedure, but I have known many children whose happiness and self-confidence have been immeasurably enhanced by it. One mother reported that her five-year-old son said when he recovered from the operation, "Now I'm like everybody else."

Paying your Bills

As with most cosmetic surgery, your surgeon's fee will probably be payable in advance. If the otoplasty is done under a local anesthesia, its cost will very likely be included in that fee. If it is done with a general anesthesia, it will mean that a trained anesthesiologist will administer the anesthetic. His bill, separate from that of your surgeon's, will probably be given to you before you leave the hospital.

The Otoplasty Technique

When ears protrude, it is most often because the fold of elastic cartilage that bends the ear towards the head is badly formed or poorly developed. The basic technique for correcting this condition goes back over a hundred years, although there are now more than a dozen different variations on it. The particular one used by a surgeon in any given case depends on his experience, personal preference, and evelution of the individual's problem. Basically, however, the otoplasty operation involves incising and removing strips of the underlying cartilage and stitching the ear into a better position in relation to the side of the head.

The incision is made on the back of the hidden surface of the ear, which makes the resulting scar invisible unless searched for. Through this incision, the skin is elevated from the underlying cartilage framework of the ear. The cartilage is then literally carved and sculpted into a more normal shape. In those cases where ridges and convolutions are missing, they are surgically fabricated and stitched in place. A small amount of excess skin is then trimmed away, and the incision is sewn tightly together to help hold the ear in its new position.

Anyone contemplating a corrective procedure for protruding ears should know that both ears will not look *exactly* the same after surgery. They hardly ever do, in the first place.

The surgical procedure lasts about an hour, and the recovery period is two to three weeks.

AFTER THE SURGERY

Bandages — Immediately after surgery, the head is snugly bandaged like a football helmet and left that way for several days to help keep the ear in its new place. When the bandage is removed, a protective wrap-around bandage or stocking cap is worn at night for a few weeks until the healing is secure. Neither adults nor children seem to mind this at all.

Pain; swelling — There is very little pain connected with an otoplasty, although there is likely to be some minor postoperative discomfort, which can be managed with mild pain medication containing no aspirin.

Moderate swelling, lasting a few weeks, is to be expected. Some discoloration in the operated area will remain for approximately a month.

Stitches and scars — Stitches are removed as an office procedure, ten days after the operation. This is painless and is often done by the surgeon's nurse.

Scarring is minimal, and because of the location of the incision, such scars as there are cannot be seen unless looked for. Unless someone knew you before the otoplasty, there is no way to detect (without an examination of the area back of your ears) that you ever had protruding ears.

The Possibility of Complications

In simple cases of protruding ears, postoperative complications are exceedingly rare. In fact, the success rate of this particular procedure is very high. Nonetheless, there is a small percentage of cases in which a second, minor corrective surgical procedure becomes necessary. While it does not occur often, an accumulation of blood under the skin sometimes has to be removed ("evacuated"). Usually, this is done as an office procedure, unless the condition arises in a hospitalized patient who has not yet been discharged.

Infection after otoplasty is also exceedingly rare, but when it occurs, it's treated with appropriate antibiotics.

Some, but very few, people develop excessive scar tissue (keloids) in the incisions. Nature causes that type of healing in certain people — it has nothing to do with the procedure or the surgeon's skill — but the number of children likely to develop keloids after an otoplasty is very small indeed. When they occur, they are treated by the injection of cortisonelike drugs (steroids) into the scar tissue. Most often, however, the keloid scars subside of their own accord.

In a small percentage of patients — perhaps 3 to 5 percent — the original condition can recur, either partially or completely, because the stitches placed to hold the cartilage in its new sculpted shape have let go. Secondary corrective procedures in such situations are almost uniformly successful.

Other Ear Imperfections

Occasionally, someone will be born with the opposite of protruding ears — the angle formed between the base of the ear and the side of the head is less than average and the ears appear to be leaning flat against the skull. Few people ever come to a surgeon asking to have this altered.

Because they are so exposed and prominent, the ears are often subject to injury in car and industrial accidents, in the boxing ring, and even from frostbite and chronic infections that can occur in pierced ears. In some cultures, biting off a piece of the ear is a favorite expression of anger. We're all familiar with the "cauliflower ear" so common among fighters. Its name is quite descriptive. This deformity, the result of blows or pounding on the ears, which causes blood clots and chronic swelling, is difficult to correct.

Then we have the "lop ear," where the top seems to fold down and forward. A "cupped ear" appears as cup-shaped, although its only real flaw is that it's too small. "Shell ears" resemble seashells — they are without the natural folds and creases

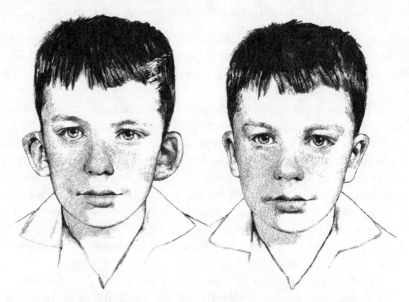

Surgical correction of a protruding ear deformity in a young boy who had been unable to camouflage his problem with long hair.

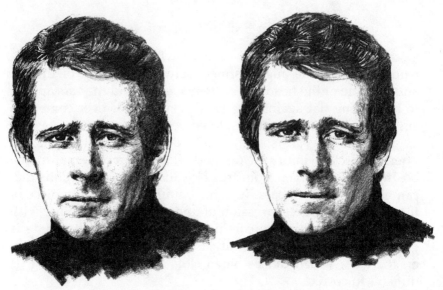

Adults often admit to emotional distress suffered since childhood because of protruding ears. Adulthood is not too late for an otoplasty, or "ear pinback," that can correct both the anatomical and emotional problems.

that most of us have. They are also missing the outer curve of the ear's rim. The "satyr ear" has a pointed tip on the top — a characteristic that caused its bearers much grief in eras of intense superstition when satyr ears were thought to be identifying marks of lascivious demigods.

Some of these abnormalities occur on both sides of the head; some affect only one ear. Occasionally, the same disfigurement will be found on both sides, but in different degrees. Sometimes a person is born with an outer ear partially or totally absent. Statistically, this happens in one out of 6,000 births, and when it occurs it does not necessarily mean that the person's inner ear is affected. It's possible to hear even if the outer ear is missing. In some people the ear canal is absent while the inner ear is present.

There are still other cosmetic ear problems. Sometimes the earlobes are too large for the ears or abnormal in the way they are attached to the head. Or the skin and tissue of the earlobes have become stretched out of shape or unduly elongated from the constant wearing of heavy earrings. This condition is more common in other cultures. It is traditional in many tribes of East Africa to pierce the ears of small children with a small wooden peg. The small pegs are replaced with larger and larger ones until the remaining earlobe is a large loop into which can be fitted and carried any number of containers with portable goodies such as snuff, tobacco, medicines, or jewelry — a handy "natural pocket" for people without pockets in their clothing. On my annual visits to Africa, I have seen tobacco tins and objects as large as baseballs carried this way. Looped earlobes were once a formal dress procedure for native colonial troops.

Sometimes, the earlobes in aging people will have multitudinous creases and wrinkles, a telltale sign of age. Wrinkled earlobes are particularly eyecatching in women who have had aesthetic facial surgery such as facelifts or chemical peels, resulting in facial skin that is relatively unwrinkled — except for the shriveled and lined earlobes.

Most of these flaws and deformities can be helped by cosmetic surgery. Some improvement can usually be made without much risk or expenditure of time and money. Stretched earlobes can be reduced even in middle age and later, and the creases of old age can be diminished by dermabrasion or chemabrasion.

Reconstruction of wholly or partially missing ears is, of course, another matter. This is one of the most complicated and difficult procedures in plastic surgery. Its complexity can be grasped if you look at the intricate folds, grooves, ridges, and angles of the human ear. Even a sculptor working in clay or wood finds it hard to do justice to this natural piece of art. For a surgeon, sculpting an ear out of living tissue takes the highest degree of skill, artistry, patience, and perseverance.

When a major portion of the ear must be replaced, a copy of the cartilage of the ear must first be prepared and then carved from a suitable piece of actual cartilage taken from the rib cage. If the patient has enough skin where the ear will go, this cartilage is then implanted beneath it. Otherwise, a skin graft or flap must be used to cover the framework of the cartilage. Implants of silicone or other synthetic materials are also used by some surgeons, but these are not always well tolerated by the body.

There is another cosmetically effective method of ear replacement that consists of fashioning an external prosthesis made of polyvinyl or other synthetic materials. This is then artfully painted and colored to match the patient's skin tone. While a perfectly sculpted and color-matched prosthesis that can be glued to the side of the head might seem the ideal solution to the problem of an absent ear, there are difficulties that preclude this alternative for many patients. To begin with, the technique is extremely difficult and the technology by no means standardized, so there are very few centers in the U.S., or anywhere else, for that matter, where truly convincing artificial ears can be obtained. Furthermore, the glues available for this purpose are unreliable and sometimes irritating to the skin. Many patients consider this more of a nuisance than they care to put up with. Also, as one's skin color changes with aging and exposure to the sun, so must the color of the prosthesis. Finally, these prostheses are quite expensive and must be replaced periodically.

Because it is so complicated a procedure, some surgeons concentrate on ear reconstruction — obviously, it is not something that can be done on an occasional basis by any cosmetic surgeon. I should speak of "procedures," because several operations are required over a period of time, the first usually at the age of four or five. Despite all this, there are quite a few plastic surgeons both in the U.S. and abroad who are able to reconstruct total ears so that they look like the real thing. Dr. Burt Brent of Stanford University in California specializes entirely in ear reconstruction and has contributed enormously to the development of this technique.

Myths about Protruding Ears — and about Ear Surgery

Some parents and patients still harbor the impression that protruding ears can result from pulling on the ears of an infant or small child, or from their being stretched as a result of lying on a "folded" ear during sleep. Certainly no normal parent would be guilty of pulling on a child's ear severely enough or often enough to create such a drastic effect, and, while pulling on one's own ear can be a habit, it certainly could not result in a protruding ear. Nor can sleeping on a "folded" ear cause it to protrude.

The most common and persistent myth is that protruding ears can be corrected by plastering them to the side of the head in infants or children with spirit gum, glue, bandages, or tape. No amount of forcing the ear to the side of the head will correct the basic problem because there is an inherited, architectural deficiency or malformation of the cartilage, and *that* has to be corrected in order for the ears to lie in place properly.

Another old wives' tale says that large ears can be reduced in size by cutting "a piece of pie" out of them. Generally, operations designed to reduce a large but normal-shaped ear are not very successful. The scars that result from such attempts are usually more noticeable than the large ear was in the first place. It is not really the size of one's ear that is noticeable to other people — it is the degree to which it protrudes. When the angle of protrusion is corrected, the ear no longer appears too large.

Unfortunately, correction of protruding or deformed ears will not eliminate the characteristic from future generations any more than a rhinoplasty will assure that someone's children or grandchildren will have a nose as lovely as the one that has been reshaped through cosmetic surgery. A cosmetic operation does not affect the genetic makeup of an individual.

I mentioned that the ears are fully grown at an earlier age than other parts of the body. Because many people believe that the ears grow until puberty, they postpone surgery until the teen years. There is really no justification for denying corrective surgery to small children who suffer the adverse psychological effects of protruding ears.

Happiness Is a Thing Called Otoplasty

The benefits of this operation are psychological as well as physical. Everyone, including the patient, quickly grows accustomed to the new look of the ears after otoplasty, and I have known young adults who, after undergoing this operation in childhood, looked at old pictures of themselves and were amazed at what they saw. "I don't remember ever looking like that" is a very common reaction. As for children whose ears embarrassed them — I can think of few things as gratifying as the comments of such children after recovery from otoplasty. "Terrific!" and "I like it, I like it!" and "I can't fly now, except in an airplane" are typical of the things small boys have been heard to say when the surgeon hands them a mirror and says, "Would you like to look in the mirror?"

Though I have emphasized otoplasty in children, this is also a procedure that makes for happiness in adults who did not have the opportunity to correct their protruding ears during their childhood. Such people, who may have been unhappy with the look of their ears for two or three decades, are often among the most satisfied patients when they finally are rid of this disturbing flaw in their appearance.

Judy came to my office some years ago when she was thirty-two, a very unhappy woman who complained that her ears were like teacup handles and that her parents had done her a grave injustice by not having them corrected when she was young. She had never married and was despondent because she had just ended a relationship with a lover of many years. She worked in the Boston headquarters office of a large insurance firm. She was a pleasant-looking woman, not a great beauty but prettier than average. Although she was about five foot five, she seemed shorter because her posture and carriage were poor, almost as though she wanted to shrink into herself and hide from the world. She struck me as the type of person who had difficulty entering a room full of people and would rather slink into it backwards. On two different occasions, when she came to my office for consultations, she was dressed in brown, without a single bit of color or jewelry.

Judy told me that her ears were "ugly" and "conspicuous" and that she felt people stared at them when talking to her. She had great difficulty, she said, finding a satisfactory hairstyle to camouflage her problem. Her ears did, indeed, protrude conspicuously, but I felt that I could correct this physical problem, especially since it meant so much to her.

The otoplasty procedure was quick, simple, and successful. She was enormously pleased with the result, and within a few months began to wear her hair brushed back off her face. She told me this was a "first" for her, and she loved it. She also changed her style of dress, appearing in more colorful and chic outfits. She began to wear earrings. I haven't seen her in years, but when last I saw her, I had the feeling that even her bearing had changed for the better. Certainly the smile on her face as she said goodbye to me after our last postoperative consultation made her look like a different person.

"I'm not self-conscious about meeting people, any more," she told me at that time. "I can actually feel relaxed in the presence of strangers. In fact, I've told my company I want to get out of the office and try my hand at sales. I think I'll be very good at it. I don't have trouble starting a conversation and people seem to like me. I know that I feel much more positive towards people than I did before. Is it possible that my ears were such a handicap they held me back? Anyway, I'm doing a lot better these days, any way you look at it. I got rid of a major hangup in my life."

"A large head of hair makes the handsome more graceful."
— Ascribed to LYCURGUS

Hair Transplants | 13

I'M NOW THIRTY-SIX, but my baldness started when I was only twenty. It was a family trait, my father and all my uncles going bald very early. Two of my uncles never married and I wouldn't be surprised if it was because they were so self-conscious about their looks. They were very shy. I was very depressed when I saw that I was balding so early in life. "Here we go," I thought, "my uncles all over again."

You can't imagine what it's like to be very young and to look in the mirror when you shave every day and know it's going to be like that, or worse, for the rest of your life. I can't tell you what it did to me. Some men can carry off baldness, but I became very self-conscious. It got worse and worse. I had something like a horseshoe effect, very bald on top, with a good ring of hair around the sides and very thick, strong hair at the back, the lower back part.

I was raised in Montreal, and I went back there for the surgery because I heard there was an excellent dermatologist who did transplants. He said I had typical male-pattern baldness and that it was due to my genes, not to any illness because, as he pointed out, the hair on the rest of my body was not affected.

He and another doctor worked on me. They did fifty plugs and it took almost two hours. The following year I went back and had another fifty done. I'm well satisfied with the results because now I can sweep some of the side hair over the plugged area and it gives the impression of a full head of hair. I plan to have another fifty done, and I will when I have the time and money. It's definitely worth it.

It satisfied my vanity. I also think the girls like my looks better, too. I just don't think young girls like to go out with bald men; at least, it's not their first choice. We all know the accent in this country is on youth and good looks, and people in general go on diets and do exercise because they want to look their best. I'm no different from anyone else; that's really all I want — to look my best. I'm happier when I look good. Why should I go through life bald when I can have hair?

Every man and nearly every woman experiences hair loss as they grow older, only the degree varies, and it varies greatly depending upon heredity, hormones, and a number of other factors. In men this process begins much earlier, sometimes when they are still in their twenties. In women, the process is slow in developing and usually begins, if at all, after the menopause.

Generally speaking, men are extremely sensitive about their hair loss, a good head of hair being associated in many minds with youthfulness, virility, and strength. To some, baldness signifies the passing of their youth, and nothing seems to assuage their feeling of dismay when they note the ebb tide of their hairline. Despite the fact that many famous men have been bald, including such symbols of virility as Yul Brynner, Telly Savalas, and Dwight D. Eisenhower, there are few balding men who do not yearn for, and often search for, some remedy that will help reverse or stem the fallout of their hair.

The pattern that baldness usually takes in men is referred to as *male-pattern baldness* and, to some degree, it affects about 95 percent of all white adult men. Such baldness is characterized by a receding hairline above the temples and forehead, with or without a bald spot at the back of the head. In women, the problem is comparatively minor, and what hair loss there is can be easily concealed, because the hair that remains can be grown longer and coiffed to successfully disguise the bald areas. Women with a severe degree of baldness resort to wigs much earlier than do most men, thus hiding their baldness as soon as it becomes noticeable.

Anatomy of the Hair

In order to understand why baldness occurs, it helps to have a basic knowledge of hair anatomy. The hair itself is known as the hair *shaft* and it grows out of the hair's *root,* a tiny tunnel embedded in fat. The root is also known as the hair *follicle.* The root, or follicle, is the buried part of the hair, invisible when you look at your scalp. If the hair shaft is damaged, it will fall out and new hair will replace it sooner or later — *provided the follicle has remained intact and healthy.* But if the follicle, imbedded in the skin, is damaged, and if that damage is irreversible, no new hair will grow out of it. When a large number of roots are irreversibly damaged, an area of baldness results.

The medical name for baldness is *alopecia,* and it is caused by two major factors: first and foremost, a hereditary tendency; second, hormonal influences. There are, in addition, a number of other possible causes of hair loss, including injury to either the root or shaft, burns, scar tissue (in which hair doesn't grow), certain infections, and some specific diseases that can produce temporary or permanent alopecia.

Prominent among the hormonal causes are thyroid and pituitary disturbances, as well as diabetes. Chemotherapy and exposure to radiation and certain chemicals can also cause alopecia, as can trauma, psychiatric and nutritional problems, poisons (toxins), drugs, and certain skin disorders.

By far the most common cause of hair loss is an imbalance in the way the body produces androgens, the male hormone that affects secondary sex characteristics such as the beard, fat distribution, and the size of the hands, feet, and muscles. Contrary to popular belief, androgens are produced in both men and women, but women produce much smaller amounts. Hair loss due to androgen activity is, naturally, called *androgenetic alopecia,* and it occurs only in people who are genetically predisposed to it. You might say that each individual hair follicle is programmed by its genetic makeup — perhaps a single dominant gene — to respond or not respond to the influences of certain substances, including androgens, that could inhibit its normal growth.

Androgenetic alopecia is very prevalent among Caucasians — about a third of all white men are affected by it to a major degree, while 95 percent suffer it to a minor extent. It is less common among Africans and relatively rare among Asians.

Apart from surgery, there are many methods of treating baldness, depending upon the cause. These include hormonal therapy, massage, treatment of specific skin disorders, and steroid injections. Surgery is frequently the choice of people who are genetically programmed for baldness and cannot be helped in any other way. Since this book is about plastic surgery and not about other treatment methods, I'm going to tell you only about that cosmetic remedy.

When alopecia occurs in small, circumscribed areas or patches, it is called alopecia *areata* (Latin for *localized*). Most such cases are reversible; that is, the hair will grow back when the underlying cause — often unknown — has disappeared. Treatment can sometimes speed the recovery period but with or without treatment (injection of steroids), this condition has a promising prognosis and does not call for surgery.

By contrast, male-pattern alopecia is usually characterized by an atrophy of the hair follicles, and despite what some charlatans claim, no remedy exists that will reverse it. There is hardly a field where the quack-remedy industry has had more willing and unquestioning customers. The truth is that until the recent advent of successful hair transplants, it was simply not possible to alter one's baldness beyond the use of a wig or hairpiece. These may be expedient for people in show business or in the public eye, but for more intimate occasions they are, at best, awkward and sometimes subject the wearer to unpleasant mishaps.

Quite recently, a drug used to reduce blood pressure was found to have an "undesirable" side effect: it made hair grow, stimulating quiescent hair follicles. This drug has been abandoned as a blood pressure remedy but is being studied as a possible treatment for baldness. (I will discuss this new drug later on in the chapter.)

Candidates for Hair Transplants

Practically every man who is greatly distressed by his loss of hair and who feels that his baldness interferes with his happiness is a candidate for hair transplants. As with every surgical procedure, one has to weigh carefully the advantages of this operation against the sacrifices it will call for in terms of time, money, and discomfort. A strong point in favor of this procedure is that, nowadays, the effectiveness is nearly always good and the risk factor that exists in all surgery is minimal in this one. If there are no medical or psychological contraindications for the surgery, hair transplants are usually successful in cases of the common, irreversible, male pattern alopecia.

BEFORE THE SURGERY

Photographs Some, but not all, doctors ask that medical photographs be taken by a medical photographer, or perhaps the doctor will take them himself. These are not designed to flatter you. They are meant for use by the physician before the operation so he can carefully study the exact location on your head where he plans to place the transplanted scalp.

Preoperative blood tests As with any elective surgery, the general health of the patient has to be assessed. This assessment usually incudes preoperative blood counts and blood chemistry in a search for any possible medical contraindications, such as poorly controlled diabetes.

Scalp preparation You will probably be told to wash your hair and scalp with an antiseptic shampoo or solution before coming in for the surgery. Some surgeons arrange for this to be done when you arrive at the treatment location.

Anesthesia A local anesthesia is always used in hair transplants. This will numb your scalp during the operation. However, the administering of the anesthesia, which is injected with a needle, can, in itself, be quite uncomfortable. To minimize this discomfort, the skin areas will first be cooled with an ethyl chloride spray that raises the threshold of pain. The nervous or apprehensive patient is well advised to take some Valium or other sedative before surgery and should ask the doctor for a prescription for such a drug if he thinks he'll need it. Pain during the actual operation is minimal. Some patients say they feel a small amount of pain or discomfort, while others report that the discomfort is not enough to warrant mentioning.

Medication   Your surgeon will give you an instruction sheet when you schedule your transplant procedure. Most such instructions include a precaution against taking aspirin or aspirin-containing compounds for one or two weeks preceding surgery and for a week afterwards. Drugs containing aspirin include Alka-Seltzer, Anacin, Bufferin, Coricidin, Darvon Compound, Dristan, Excedrin, Fiorinal, Percodan, and others. It is a known fact that aspirin inhibits the normal blood clotting mechanism. You will also be told to keep away from alcohol for several days prior to and after surgery, since alcohol tends to increase swelling.

Where surgery is performed   Hair transplant operations are performed on an outpatient basis, usually in the doctor's office or in a special clinic facility he has set up for this type of surgery.

Length of procedure   The length of the procedure depends, of course, on how much transplanting is being done. On the average, a transplant session will last one to two hours.

Paying your bill   As with all cosmetic surgery, you will probably be asked to pay the doctor's fee before the procedure is performed, or upon leaving the office or clinic after surgery. You will want to check your medical policies, but the likelihood is that the procedure is *not* covered by your medical insurance.

Hair Transplant Techniques

The surgical treatment of baldness can be done in three ways, the choice depending upon the preference of the doctor performing the transplant and upon where, on the head, the patient still has a good growth of hair.

The first of these procedures, the one used most frequently, involves a "free" graft of hair to a bald area from another place on the head where the hair still grows. The word "free" refers to the fact that the hair and its root (or follicle) are surgically "freed" from their original growth area, lifted out, and then planted elsewhere, much as you would transplant a bulb from one place in the ground to another. In the second type of procedure, a flap of hair-bearing skin is rotated or flapped over to another area where no hair is growing. In this procedure, the piece of normal scalp tissue bearing the healthy hair and follicle is not severed but remains attached to the head by means of a *pedicle* (or stalk of skin) that is going to be redraped to another site. In such cases, the shafts and roots continue to be nourished by blood vessels running through the pedicle. The third procedure is one in which a whole strip of scalp, bearing healthy hair, is moved to another part of the head.

How a Free Graft Works

The technique of grafting tiny areas of hairy scalp tissue onto bald spots was pioneered in the late fifties by Dr. Norman Orentreich, a New York City dermatologist. His procedure, or variations of it, is being used all over the world with excellent results. The operation consists of removing a small plug of skin containing a complete individual hair shaft in its follicle from the hair-bearing part of the scalp. This plug is removed with a sharp, small, round surgical gouge or punch, usually operated by hand, although some surgeons use a motorized version of this tool.

The small graft can be likened to a divot of sod that can be raised by a golf club, except that it is perfectly round. The plug is taken from an area of the scalp that is rich in hair and not involved in the balding process. This is known as the *donor area*. Each small wound created in the donor area is either left open to heal naturally or closed with a small stitch. Eventually, all that will remain will be a small scar. (In the case of patients who have suffered loss of hair from severe burns and loss of scalp skin, hair-bearing skin grafts can be transferred from elsewhere on the body, such as the pubic region. These free grafts require microsurgery to sew together the very small blood vessels needed to nourish the transplanted area.)

The hair-bearing plug, after being cleaned, trimmed of excess tissue, fat, and loose hair, is then transferred to an area of baldness, usually in the front or very top of the head. The implantation is done in the same way: the identical round cutting tool is used to remove a plug of bald skin that is the same size as the grafted plug. The grafted plug is then sutured into place with one or two minute stitches or simply taped into place with paper surgical tape. The hairless plug of recipient skin is discarded.

Almost all of these grafts survive as "takes." They heal in place and become nourished by the blood vessels of the recipient scalp and by new blood vessels that grow into the graft. The hairs themselves don't always survive the transfer, however, since there is a period during the healing process when the nutrition provided to the hair follicle by the blood vessels is marginal; or, at best, minimal. If the hair follicle housing the shaft is not a healthy one when transplanted, the prognosis for its survival is not good. But if the hair and root are hardy, they can usually withstand this minor injury to their health and remain unaffected by hormones, aging, or genetic tendencies to hair loss.

Even under the best of circumstances, actual hair growth cannot be expected for the first three months after the procedure. Initially, after the operation, it may appear that the hair in the grafts is growing. Most of the transplanted shafts are, in fact, usually in the process of falling out. This is a normal occurrence. Those that regrow do so after a period of three weeks to three months.

Transplanting hair by the plug technique usually requires

several sessions. The average scalp has about 100,000 hairs. Each skin plug to be transplanted measures less than a sixth of an inch in diameter and holds about ten to fifteen hairs. Transplanting 500 or 1,000 plugs would provide a good head of hair, although most people settle for 200 to 300 plugs, which are adequate for good cosmetic results.

Ten to sixty plugs are usually transplanted in each session, although some doctors do as many as a hundred. On the average, one must figure anywhere between three to five such sessions, although many patients are quite satisfied with the results of two or three, performed over a period of several months. The actual number transplanted in a single session depends on the doctor's speed, the patient's tolerance for the procedure, and the amount of hair to be transplanted.

About 99 percent of the transplanted skin plugs will eventually produce hair. While the operation itself is not difficult, the skill of the surgeon is a major factor in determining the end result. It takes good judgment to choose the proper hair for removal and the right location for the graft. It is also important for the doctor to observe the direction in which the patient's hair normally grows so that he can correctly position the skin plugs in the punched-out holes. Otherwise, the newly implanted hair could grow randomly in various directions. This would make hair coiffing very difficult.

Mark, a young stockbroker who had just turned thirty, had complained that his shortness (he was five foot four) combined with baldness, "put two strikes against" him. He said he wanted to "fight nature, if at all possible and give myself a break in life." He was ecstatic over the results of 100 plugs transplanted during a two-year period. He said to his doctor, "You're tall. You have lots of hair. Can you imagine what it was like for me to be so doubly cheated by nature? I'm really very happy about the difference it's made in my looks. It's just like my own hair — because it *is* my own hair. I'd recommend it for anyone who needs it and can afford it. It's nothing to be afraid of."

The Flap-Over

Another successful method of treating baldness surgically was devised by an Argentinean, Dr. José Juré. This technique calls for the replacement of bald areas with hair-bearing skin flaps.

It requires an island of full-thickness skin, which is growing healthy hair and located in sufficient proximity to the recipient area, so it can be flapped over or rotated into position to provide hairbearing scalp to a bald region. The pedicle, or connecting link between the old site and the new one, forms the conduit through which the blood vessels can provide continuing nourishment to the transplanted piece of scalp.

The Strip Graft

For reconstructing the hairline along the front of the scalp, Dr. Charles Vallis of Boston modified the punch graft technique so that the entire front line of hair can be restored by grafting a single strip of hairbearing scalp, rather than using multiple punches. In this procedure, a strip of healthy scalp approximately one-quarter inch in width is taken from the back of the head and transplanted into an incision placed exactly along the frontal line at the top of the forehead where the normal hairline would be. With this technique, it is even possible to create a widow's peak.

After the front line of the scalp is established with such a strip graft, the remaining baldness behind the line can be filled in with punch grafts or even with a series of strip grafts laid in a row.

Mostly, however, the punch graft method is the operation of choice because the risk of rejection of the graft increases as the size of the graft increases. Furthermore, with larger grafts, the scars formed at the donor site are likely to be more visible.

HAIR WEAVING . . . NOT RECOMMENDED HERE

There is yet another surgical procedure for treating baldness by means of hair implantation. It is known as *hair weaving*, and I must state unequivocally that I do not recommend it.

In this form of surgery, threads made of Teflon-coated wire are woven into the scalp with a needle. These threads are then used to attach hand-woven hairpieces that match the patient's own hair in color. The end result is a substitute for a removable type of hairpiece and is touted by those who perform the procedure as being much better than wigs, or even other surgeries, because the implants are seemingly well anchored into the skin.

However, it is a medically unsatisfactory procedure because the body tends to reject the implant of these foreign bodies and because of the frequency of infections. The Food and Drug Administration has determined that the weaving of artificial hair elements into the scalp is unsafe and ineffective; it strongly condemns this method.

Selecting Your Doctor

Many, though not all, plastic surgeons do hair transplants. There are also many dermatologists who are qualified to perform these procedures, and some make it their major subspecialty. The flap-over and strip graft procedures are, however, almost always performed by plastic surgeons. (As I mentioned before, the free graft or plug method was pioneered by a dermatologist.) Whichever of the three procedures is the one you will undergo, you should be certain that your doctor has had extensive experience in this type of operation.

While some commercial, nonmedical salons exist for the purpose of doing hair transplants, I would be reluctant to choose any of them over a qualified doctor. Despite the seeming simplicity of the procedure, judgment and a knowledge of anatomy are called for in selecting donor sites, in deciding the best distance between implants, and in monitoring the small amount of bleeding that can be expected whenever surgery is performed. Because baldness is so distressing to so many people, it offers ample opportunity for the unscrupulous to profit at the expense of unsuspecting and uninformed persons. I would urge you not to submit to any form of surgical treatment — and that includes hair transplants — except at the hands of a qualified doctor.

The best ways to find a medical specialist in hair transplantation are to ask your internist, your plastic surgeon, or your dermatologist, if you have one; to call the local medical society for a referral; or to ask a friend who has successfully undergone the procedure himself and can recommend his doctor.

Sometimes a dermatologist or plastic surgeon will reject a request for hair transplanting because he feels the patient is not realistic enough about his expectations for the procedure; or if the process of hair loss is insufficiently advanced for the doctor to be able to see whether the problem will be minor or severe, or where the best donor and recipient sites might be. In such cases, the doctor will often say, "Let's wait," meaning that it's in your own best interests to let the problem establish itself fully before taking any surgical action.

As with all cosmetic surgery, realistic expectations for the procedure make for successful results and happy patients. If you discuss a hair transplant with a physician, it is important that you come away from the consultation with a clear picture of what such surgery can do for you — and what it cannot do. Someone who expects that 50 plugs, inserted in a free graft transplant procedure, will promote a full and bushy head of hair is going to be disappointed with the actual results of the surgery. It is perfectly appropriate for you to inquire, in a consultation, what the doctor believes the end result of the surgery will be.

AFTER THE SURGERY

Bandages

After the surgery, your head will very likely be treated with an antibiotic ointment and bandaged to minimize swelling (edema). This dressing will be removed in approximately 24 hours.

Discomfort, bleeding, and scarring

Rarely does anyone experience postoperative pain. However, when the local anesthetic wears off, you may well experience some discomfort in both the donor and recipient sites. Your doctor will probably prescribe medication to minimize whatever discomfort you are likely to feel. Or he may suggest you take something as mild as Tylenol, which contains no aspirin.

Occasionally, there is some postoperative bleeding, particularly if the scalp is accidentally scratched. While you should report any bleeding to your doctor or his nurse, it is likely to disappear by the second day.

The small crusts that form around each

graft are part of the healing process — they are, in effect, nature's own bandages. They must not be picked at.

Exercise There should be no strenuous exercise for at least a week after the operation. This includes jogging, tennis, or any sport that requires you to jump off the ground, such as basketball or volleyball. If you need to lift anything heavy, do so by bending at the knees.

THE POSSIBILITY OF COMPLICATIONS

Hair transplanting is a procedure in which complications are rare; if they occur, they are usually of a minor and self-curing nature. Swelling of the forehead down to the eyebrows can occur, but it is a temporary condition that does not require treatment. Some patients have a black eye (sometimes two!) within a day after surgery, but this, too will disappear without treatment.

While infections and keloid (heavy scarring) formations can occur, both are quite rare. A slight feeling of numbness at the graft sites is not uncommon and can last for weeks or even months. But this, too, is nothing to worry about — a small price to pay for the physical and emotional rewards that usually follow this procedure.

A LOOK AT THE FUTURE

One of the great pluses of hair transplants is that the results last. In fact, once it begins to grow, the newly grafted hair is there to stay, at least as long as all the other hair that remains in the donor sites. The pleasure of seeing hair grow again where none would grow before is of inestimable value. Of course, it may take a while to see the final results and, along the way, the newly transplanted hair may fall out before a new growth appears. But once it *does* start to grow, the transplanted hair is all *yours* — grown from your own roots, in your own scalp; you can comb it, cut it, and brush it and — best of all — it will not fall out.

Transplant patients, if they undergo the procedure with a good understanding of what they can expect, are among the most satisfied of all patients who seek cosmetic surgery. Perhaps the people most pleased with their hair transplants are those in public life — people on television, in show business, in government or politics, as well as those in education and the business world. In addition to the professional advantages that accrue under certain circumstances when men are thought to be young or in the prime of life, is the enhanced self-image that people report after successful hair transplants.

The Promise of a New, Helpful Drug

One of the most exciting pieces of recent news has to do with a new drug, produced for other purposes, that holds out some promise as a cure for baldness. However, we must, as of now, approach reports about this drug with considerable caution because there is insufficient proof of its efficacy for this purpose; and knowledge about possible side effects is far from complete.

The drug is called *minoxidil*, and it was introduced a few years ago for the treatment of severe hypertension (high blood pressure). When it was found that hair appeared to grow on some, but not all, of the people who had been put on this drug, there was a good deal of public enthusiasm and encouragement to establish minoxidil as a treatment for hair loss. But though the drug had been thoroughly researched as a hypertension medication and released by the FDA for *that* purpose, the research on its use as a treatment for baldness has not been going on long enough for all the facts, including possible side effects, to have become clear.

The drug is now being studied, both in lotion and ointment form, to find out if it can be cosmetically acceptable as a partial or total remedy for baldness. The evidence thus far appears to indicate that the results are better with people who suffer patchy, rather than total, alopecia.

At the time of this writing, the bad news is that there is evidence of unpleasant side effects in some people for whom this drug has been prescribed. Such side effects seem to consist primarily of local skin irritations. But many other factors are, as yet, unknown: what percentage of individuals will respond to treatment with minoxidil if prescribed for alopecia? How many will suffer unpleasant side effects? And will the hair growth —

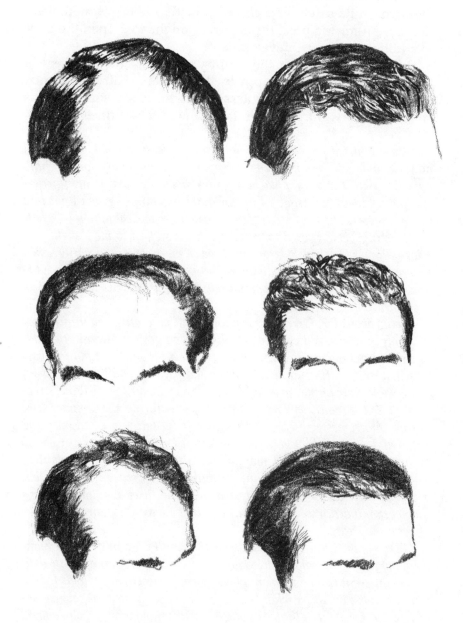

Illustrations above show various types of baldness patterns. On the right, results that can be achieved by hair-bearing transplants.

if there is any — be temporary or permanent? So, before the FDA will recommend minoxidil for this purpose, much more research on its safety and efficacy must be done. Nonetheless, this is a promising breakthrough that might well open the door to additional product development.

Meanwhile, all over the country, fairly sizable numbers of patients are being made happy by the results of hair transplants. A Midwestern university professor had this to say some months after he underwent punch graft treatment for baldness.

I'm a tenured professor, I'm only forty-seven years old, so this had nothing to do with my job being in jeopardy because of age, or anything related to that. Actually, I had been going bald since I was in my thirties, and the baldness had troubled me for quite some time. When I got into my midforties, I began to notice that I no longer looked young — whatever "young" is supposed to be today. But it seemed to me I might look a lot younger if I had hair on my head. One is aware of aging when surrounded by so many really young people, all my students. My hairline had receded so badly that I grew heavy sideburns as a form of compensation.

I read about Dr. Orentreich's punch graft procedure and it intrigued me. Suffice it to say, I couldn't let it go once I got the idea in my head. When I saw a doctor in consultation, I felt a bit silly, actually embarrassed at my vanity. But he told me he had patients of all ages, in every conceivable walk of life, who felt the same way about their baldness that I did. I had three transplant procedures, one during the summer, one during intersemester break, and another at Eastertime. I had over 150 grafts and while I think a very sophisticated person, were he or she to examine my scalp, would know my hair up front's been transplanted, I don't think the average person, certainly not my students, could tell, if they cared enough to be interested. My wife likes it a lot. She says she never minded my baldness but now that I have this hair, she thinks it's simply great.

Personally, I feel very good about the results. I don't think anyone would choose to be bald. I chose not to be — nothing wrong with that. It's no different from a woman who is born a brunette and turns herself into a blonde; or a girl who gets her nose fixed. If medical science has progressed far enough to make something like this possible, why should I lag behind the times? The truth is that I like what I see in the mirror much better and it's boosted my spirits considerably.

Uncommon Procedures and Developing Techniques | 14

WHILE THE FACIAL COSMETIC surgery procedures I've described in this book have been employed hundreds of thousands of times on people seeking to improve their looks, sense of well-being, and the quality of their lives, there are certain other corrective surgical techniques that are used less frequently, both because there are fewer people in need of such facial surgery and because some of the techniques are relatively new. Since patients do occasionally consult with me and other surgeons about these procedures, the questions and answers that follow provide some basic facts about these techniques.

QUESTION: Is it possible to create dimples?
ANSWER: Yes, but the request to do so is rare. Since the era of Shirley Temple, many people have considered dimples to be "cute" and, sometimes, a mark of beauty. It is fortunate that few people seek to have facial dimples created, because making them by surgery is not easy. Only one technique seems to be effective.

QUESTION: What is that technique?
ANSWER: A dimple is, after all, simply a depression in the cheek. It comes and goes as the facial expression changes — it is not

always seen in the resting face. The technique for creating a reasonable facsimile of a natural dimple involves the creation of a small cone of scar tissue beneath the skin. The surgeon quite literally bores a small hole into the tissues beneath the skin. This is done from within, not externally.

Using an instrument similar to the one used in hair transplants (when a plug of healthy scalp is moved to a bald spot on the head), the surgeon punches out a small cone of normal tissue at the precise spot beneath the skin where the dimple is desired, usually in the midcheek region. This creates a small cavity in the cheek, which extends to the underside of the skin but does not go through to the outside. Thus, the scar is not visible as a skin scar.

As the tissue heals, a scar forms. It is in the nature of scar tissue to contract like a rubber band as the scar heals and matures. With such contraction, a small area of skin on the cheek is drawn inwards, resulting in a permanent depression in the cheek.

QUESTION: Does it look like a real dimple?
ANSWER: The depression created by surgery does resemble a dimple, the only difference being that it is present at all times, regardless of whether the face is at rest or is laughing, moving, or otherwise animated. Its permanence creates a slightly unnatural impression.

QUESTION: What causes "fatty cheeks"?
ANSWER: Fatty cheeks should not be confused with full faces, or high cheekbones. Just beneath the layer of muscle in each cheek is a small pad of fat. For unknown reasons — heredity probably plays a role — some people have overdeveloped ("hypertrophied") fat pads, which create very full, rounded cheeks. Earlier in this century, the heart-shaped face was considered beautiful, and people with fatty cheeks were not at all troubled by them. However, the gaunt look is more in vogue these days, and otherwise slender people, almost always women, sometimes consult a plastic surgeon because they feel that their fatty cheeks give them a chubby appearance.

QUESTION: Can anything be done to diminish or eliminate fatty cheeks?

ANSWER: True hypertrophy of these fat pads can be eliminated quite simply by removing the offending fatty bulk. Through a small incision made inside the mouth, the fat is teased out. This leaves no external scars. The operation is a delicate one, as the surgeon must exercise great care to prevent damage to the small nerves passing through the area. However, it is not considered a dangerous operation, and the results are usually excellent, with patient satisfaction running very high.

Another method employed by surgeons to remove this fat is the recently developed suction technique known as liposuction or suction lipectomy, in which a small tube (known as a "cannula"), much like a soda straw, is inserted into the middle of the fat collection and the excess fat is literally suctioned out by a suction pump.

QUESTION: Is it possible to create a cleft in the chin?
ANSWER: It can be done, but most plastic surgeons are not enthusiastic about performing this procedure. Over the years, I have had a number of requests from men to create a "Kirk Douglas chin," which some people consider a look of virility. I have performed the operation several times but have never been completely satisfied wih the results; a surgically made cleft has an artificial appearance, especially when the face muscles are in motion.

QUESTION: How is the cleft created?
ANSWER: To make a chin cleft, the surgeon must create scar tissue, for it is the attachment of such tissue to the bone of the chin that produces the cleft. An incision is made either in the mouth or underneath the chin line, where it is virtually hidden. As in the creation of a cheek dimple, a piece of tissue beneath the skin is removed, although the skin itself is neither cut through nor injured. The skin is then forced against the underlying bone and, hopefully, as the scar tissue develops, it will adhere to the bone covering (*periostium*). This attachment is permanent, and the resulting cleft is present whether the face is at rest or in motion.

QUESTION: You sound less than enthusiastic about this procedure. Am I correct?
ANSWER: Yes. I have never seen an artificially created chin cleft

that looked natural to me. If you are interested in this procedure for yourself, I would urge you to exercise caution in selecting your surgeon. I strongly recommend that you ask to see photographs of the results of such an operation performed by any surgeon who agrees to do the operation for you.

QUESTION: If lips are unattractively large or protruding, can plastic surgery do anything for them?
ANSWER: Full lips can be beautiful and sexy, depending on their contour and size and whether they are in balance with the rest of the face. But lips that are too large and protruding can be unattractive, and many people with such lips find them distressing. Enlarged lips may be due to heredity, they can be a racial characteristic, or caused by glandular or other disturbances. Often, the cause is unknown.

Requests to improve such lips are not at all uncommon and an operation called cheiloplasty (*cheilos* is the Greek word for lip) is a simple procedure, and the result is highly successful in almost all patients.

QUESTION: What's involved in the procedure?
ANSWER: A strip of excessive tissue is removed along the full length of the lip, along its inside surface. Occasionally, it is necessary to extend the incision past the corners of the mouth and into the lining of the cheeks. The incision is then sewn together. The scar that results is inside the mouth, and therefore not visible. Although one or both lips can be reduced in this manner, reduction of the lower lip is more common, particularly among Caucasians.

The operation does not affect the way the lips close and, although some swelling of the lips can occur after surgery and last for days, weeks, or even months, the great majority of patients feel that the resultant thinner lips, with no visible scars, make the procedure worthwhile.

QUESTION: Is there any way to correct a gummy smile?
ANSWER: Some people are born with the upper lip connected too high to the upper jaw, or "tethered," creating what is medically referred to as an "open lip posture." The upper central teeth are perpetually visible, much like those in a rodent, which has caused the condition to be referred to as the "Bugs Bunny syndrome."

Patients with this facial deformity may or may not be mouth breathers, but their facial expression suggests mouth breathing since the mouth is almost always open, unless the lips are forced into closure. The smile in such people can be particularly unattractive as the lips curl upward and the upper gum is exposed to create "the gummy smile."

This condition can often be improved and frequently eliminated during plastic surgery of the nose. It cannot be eliminated, however, if the principal cause is an elongated upper jaw or protruding teeth. In such cases, only surgery to the upper jaw can correct the problem. In less complicated cases, reduction of the high nasal profile and loosening of the upper lip from the underlying upper jawbone can achieve remarkable improvement.

QUESTION: Recent newspaper and magazine articles have reported that it is now possible for a surgeon, with the use of a computer, to show you beforehand exactly what changes there will be in your face after cosmetic surgery. Is this possible?

ANSWER: Perhaps, in years to come, this might be feasible, but as of now, it simply is not. The computer, as it is now being used by a handful of surgeons who like to impress potential patients with up-to-the-minute techniques, is a very expensive "marketing toy" that provides an interesting bit of wishful thinking. Patients are sometimes led to believe their cosmetic surgery will be done with "computer precision." It is, of course, quite possible to show before-and-after pictures of a face on a computer screen — it is not all that difficult to have the computer add or subtract lines and increase or diminish the size of a nose or chin.

What is *not* possible, however, is to duplicate in the operating room what was shown on the computer screen.

QUESTION: Is there any acceptable use of the computer in planning facial surgery?

ANSWER: Computer technology has been used for several years to help the physician involved in reconstructive surgery plan what he hopes to do in rebuilding complicated facial bone and skull problems due to injuries, or deformities due to birth or developmental defects. Such use of the computer is, however, still considered to be in the research or experimental stage. Furthermore, the equipment needed to do such surgical planning is extremely expensive, and operating such equipment calls for the full-time services of a research team. Special X rays, CAT scans, and other sophisticated data are also needed to feed pertinent information into the computer. In no way does this computer resemble the desk-top model you may have in your home or office, or which you've seen in your doctor's office. Only a few medical teaching centers in the world have access to the kind of equipment involved in these reconstruction planning procedures; only a small number of people are carrying on research with it at this time.

One such research center is the Institute for Reconstructive Plastic Surgery at New York University, the institution with which I am associated. But neither here, nor elsewhere, is the work sufficiently advanced to be in the realm of possibility for everyday use by plastic surgeons. Today's computerized use of CAT scan tomography is limited to guiding a surgical team in reshaping facial bones and skulls in the most highly complicated problems. And even in these instances, it is still considered a backup tool in the surgical planning stage; it has not replaced the more conventional methods of planning.

QUESTION: Do you see computers in use in the future for aesthetic facial surgery?
ANSWER: I do not rule out the possibility that computers will eventually be useful in planning the common, everyday cosmetic surgery procedure. I certainly hope they will be — and I will be first in line to use one. Right now, if you're considering facial surgery for cosmetic reasons, I must advise you not to expect a computer to play a role in your operation — or even in the planning of it.

It is not only because computers are not ready to render such services in this type of operation. There is another equally important reason why this sort of technology cannot be involved in your procedure: cosmetic operations on human flesh are not precise. The results are not totally predictable. In this book I have pointed out several times that human tissue cannot be counted on to respond precisely as we would have it — that even the sculptor working in clay or wood is better able to anticipate exact results than can a surgeon. The anatomical aspects of the problem that brings a patient to a surgeon's office, as well as his or her genetic makeup, healing power, age, skin condition, general physical health, and other factors, all determine the outcome. No computer is yet able to influence or predict these factors.

I do believe you can learn just as much about the changes to expect from surgery if your physician were to draw lines on a photograph of you. This method of "forecasting" is likely to be more accurate than lines drawn on a computer screen image.

I also believe that the gigantic strides made by computer technology in our own time indicate that almost anything is possible in the future. We should remain open-minded about the ways in which scientific and technological advances may some day guide the hand of the surgeon.

Until that day arrives, consider the vast number of people who have undergone any one of the surgical procedures described in this book, and you are bound to conclude that cosmetic surgery in the late twentieth century is capable of effecting some extraordinary changes in the human face.

More Than Just a Pretty Face | 15

F OR EVERY PERSON WHO IS CONTENT with his or her looks, there are countless others who wish that nature had blessed them with some more attractive feature: a more shapely nose, flatter ears, a stronger jaw, or possibly one that protrudes less. For every person who is proud of having aged well, there are a hundred who would like to erase or alter the imprint that time has etched on their faces.

Living in an age when people are concerned about health, fitness, and maintaining their youthfulness, such topics as low cholesterol, no-fat diets, weight watching, jogging schedules, tennis tournaments, working out, and hair coloring are very much a part of our daily conversation. Contact lenses, hidden hearing aids, cosmetic dentistry, including adult orthodontia, and hairpieces and wigs have grown enormously popular during the last decade. It was only to be expected that the subject of cosmetic surgery would, in this environment, come out of the closet and into the mainstream of our lives. People have learned that if you look better, you feel better; that physical improvement almost always leads to psychological improvement — in one's personality and sense of well-being.

There was a time, not so long ago, when people would look in the mirror, see that fate, by way of their genes, had been unkind; or that aging had taken its toll, and they would think, "This is what I am going to look like for the rest of my life." Not anymore. In recent years, altering an unappealing feature, or restoring a face to a degree of its former youthful symmetry, has worked wonders with hundreds of thousands of people.

Wanting to look more attractive, more rested, more youthful, is not a matter of mere vanity — there is no evidence that Ponce de León was a vain man. It is the modern person's way of saying, "I want to look as good as I *can* . . . as good as I *feel*." Accepted as a legitimate branch of medicine, moving ahead rapidly with new and evolving techniques, no longer the province of the rich and famous, cosmetic surgery has most assuredly come of age.

Over the years, I have found that people who undergo successful cosmetic surgery develop a new view of themselves. The person lurking inside dares to come forth. Often, their personality changes with their looks. The surgery symbolizes new beginnings and one feels an inexplicable joyousness. All of life seems to take on a new face.

These are the typical comments every plastic surgeon hears frequently from postoperative patients:

"I feel as though I'm beginning life anew."

"I have cut back on the evidence that time is passing."

"I hadn't realized that I suffered from a low-level, chronic depression. It has lifted. I am truly happy for the first time in my life."

"It was only my face that was operated on but I feel physically invigorated."

"I look alert. I look awake. I feel alive."

"It's my time and I want to make the most of it. Now I can."

"I feel more desirable."

"Now I'm the person I want to be."

Every woman who has had her hair attractively restyled and looks in the beauty parlor mirror thinking, "I like it. I look terrific," knows what a lift even a small change in appearance can give her. She leaves the shop feeling better about herself, wanting to see friends, walking a bit taller. Her body language talks.

Every plastic surgeon knows that, after full recovery from a cosmetic operation, patients almost always present themselves in a more confident manner. So, should you, too, decide at some time that one of the operations described in this book is for you, and should you undergo the procedure and achieve your realistic goals, you may be one of the many who end up with more than just a pretty — or handsome — face. It is not unlikely that such surgery will enhance your self-esteem, brighten your hopes for the future, and rekindle your sense of optimism, and that your new looks and improved self image will help you move forward in many aspects of your life.

> "Look in thy glass, and tell the face thou viewest
> Now is the time that face should form another. . . ."
>
> WILLIAM SHAKESPEARE, *Sonnets*, X

Appendix

Type of Surgery	Where Performed (Hospital/ Ambulatory)	Number of Days in Hospital	Anesthetic (Local/ General)	Length of Procedure
Facelift (Rhytidectomy)	Either	1–3	Either	2–3 hours
Eyelid Surgery (Blepharoplasty)	Either	1–2	Either	1–2 hours
Nose Surgery (Rhinoplasty)	Either	1–3	Either	½–1½ hours
Chemabrasion	Either	1–3	Either	Varies by area treated: 1–1½ hours
Dermabrasion	Either	1–3	Either	½–1 hour
Hair Transplant	Ambulatory	—	Usually local	1–2 hours each session
Silicone Injections	Ambulatory	—	None	Depends on area treated
Collagen Injections	Ambulatory	—	None	Depends on area treated
Ear Surgery	Either	1	Either	1–2 hours
Protruding Jaw	Hospital	2–3	General	2–4 hours
Chin Augmentation (Mentoplasty)	Either	1–2	Either	½–1 hour
Forehead and Brow Lift	Either	1–2	Either	1–2 hours

Bandage/Suture Removal	Scars	Number of Days until Makeup May Be Worn	Number of Days until Hair May Be Shampooed	Back to Work
Bandages: 24–48 hours Sutures: 6–10 days	Around ears and in hair, almost invisible	10	6 days; tinting and coloring: 3 weeks	2–3 weeks
Sutures: 3–5 days	Barely visible after 6 months to 1 year	10–21	3 days, with care	3 days to 3 weeks
Nasal pack: 24–48 hours Splints: 7–10 days Sutures: if present, 3–4 days	Usually none Rarely, under nostrils	After removal of splint (7–10)	After removal of splint, 7–10 days	10 days
Tape removed after 48 hours	None	14–21	2–3 days, with care	10–18 days
None	None	14–21	2–3 days, with care	10–18 days
Bandages: 24 hours	Covered by new hair	—	Next day	Immediately
—	None	12 hours after injection	Immediately	Immediately
—	None	12 hours after injection	Immediately	Immediately
Bandages: several days Sutures: 10 days	Back of ear, minimal and almost invisible	Immediately	7 days	1–7 days
Bandages: 2 days	Occasional external scar beneath jawline, each side	14	7 days	2–3 weeks
Sutures: 7 days Tape: 3–4 days	Under chin, almost invisible	14	2 days	3–10 days
Bandages: 48 hours Sutures and staples: 6–12 days	Hidden by hair	Immediately	7 days	1–2 weeks

Index

Acne scars
  collagen treatment for, 208
  dermabrasion for, 155, 156, 171–173
Adhesive mask, for chemabrasion, 165, 166–167
Aging
  effects of, 22
  eyelids and, 92–94
  facelift and, 45–46
  fear of, 7
Allergies
  collagen treatment and, 204, 206
  rhinoplasty and, 128
Alopecia. *See* Baldness
Alopecia areata, 230. *See also* Baldness
Ambulatory surgical centers, 35–37, 99–100
American Board of Plastic Surgery, 29–30
American Society of Plastic and Reconstructive Surgeons (ASPRS), 3, 30, 200
Androgens, 229
Anesthesia
  bill for, 52
  for chemabrasion, 164
  for dermabrasion, 174
  for ear surgery, 216
  for eyelid surgery, 100–101
  for facelift, 51–52
  for hair transplants, 231–232
  for jaw surgery, 80–81
  for rhinoplasty, 129–130
Artificial tear ointments and drops, 103–104
Aspirin, 48–49

Baker, Dr. Thomas, 157
Baldness
  attitudes toward, 227–228
  causes of, 229–230
  drugs for, 230, 240
  forehead and brow lift and, 187
  hair transplants for, 230–231
  male-pattern, 228–230
  patchy, 230, 240
  treating, 227–242
Bleeding
  during dermabrasion, 174
  during facelift, 48–49, 51, 56–57, 58
  during rhinoplasty, 135–136, 140
Blepharoplasty. *See* Eyelid surgery
Blindness, eyelid surgery and, 96

257

258 | INDEX

Blood coagulation
  aspirin and, 48–49
  Vitamin K and, 76
Bone cut, for chin augmentation, 75
Bone grafts, for chin augmentation, 75
Breasts, silicone injections, 199
Brow lift. *See* Forehead and brow lift
Bruising
  after eyelid surgery, 104
  after facelift, 58, 61
  after forehead and brow lift, 190
  after rhinoplasty, 134–135, 139
Bugs Bunny Syndrome, 246–247

Cauliflower ear, 219
Chemabrasion
  anesthesia for, 164
  complications, 176–178
  contraindications for, 163
  dermabrasion and, 155–156, 176
  facelift and, 158, 179
  good candidates for, 158–162
  on hands, 160
  history of, 157–158
  hospital stay for, 163–164
  itching after, 166
  medical history and, 163
  myths about, 178–179
  new skin formation after, 167, 169
  pain involved, 165, 166
  postsurgical treatments, 168
  preoperative photographs, 162
  preoperative procedures, 162–164
  recovery from, 166–169
  results of, 156–157, 180–181
  skin type and, 159–160
  summary information, 254–255
  technique for, 156, 164–165
Chemical peeling. *See* Chemabrasion
Chin augmentation, 4, 53, 73–78, 85
  allergic reaction, 82
  loss of sensation from, 81–82
  medication prior to, 76–77
  need for, 72–73
  pain and, 78
  postsurgical diet, 78
  postsurgical medication, 77–78
  postsurgical procedures, 77–78
  preoperative photographs, 76
  strapping for, 77
  summary information, 254–255
Chin cleft, creating, 245–246
Collagen treatments, 196, 199, 204–205
  allergic reaction to, 206, 207
  complications, 207–208
  external application of, 208
  injection procedure, 206–207
  myths about, 208–209
  outlook for, 209
  preoperative procedures, 205–206
  summary information, 254–255
  Zyderm Collagen, 205–207
Complexion
  chemabrasion and, 159–160
  after facelift, 58–59
Complications
  chemabrasion, 176–178
  dermabrasion, 176–178
  ear surgery, 218–219
  eyelid surgery, 108–109
  forehead and brow lift, 190–191
  hair transplants, 239
  jaw surgery, 81–82
  rhinoplasty, 140–146
Consultations, 17–31
  expectations and, 20–21
  preparing for, 21–22
  questions to ask, 24–27
Contact lenses, 107
Cosmetic surgeons
  consultation with, 17–31
  credentials of, 29–30
  fees of, 30
  relationship with, 18–19
  selecting, 15–16
  turndown of patients by, 44
Cosmetic surgery. *See also* specific types
  benefits of, 5, 251–253
  computers and, 247–249
  defined, 6
  doubts concerning, 27–28
  early secrecy regarding, 13–14
  history of, 3–6, 13–16
  limitations of, 8–10, 21
  results of, 251–253
  "secret" techniques, 14–15
  suntanning and, 179–180
Cosmetics, *See* Makeup
Craniofacial surgery, 82–85

Crow's feet, 93, 156
Cupped ear, 219

Dermabrasion, 169–176
 for acne scars, 171
 anesthesia for, 174
 bleeding during, 174
 chemabrasion and, 155–156, 176
 complications, 176–178
 crust formation after, 174–175
 vs. facelift, 179
 history of, 169–171
 hospital stay for, 173
 myths about, 178–179
 postoperative procedures, 175–176
 preoperative photogaphs, 173
 preoperative procedures, 173–174
 summary information, 254–255
 sun protection after, 176, 177
 technique for, 171, 174–175
Deviated septum, 130–131
Dimples, creating, 243–244
Discoloration. *See* Bruising

Earlobes
 imperfections in, 221
 wrinkled, 221
Ears
 artificial, 222
 cauliflower ear, 219
 cupped ear, 219
 imperfections in, 219–223
 lop ear, 219
 partially or totally missing, 221, 222–223
 protruding, 213–217, 223–224
 reconstructing, 222–223
 reducing size of, 223
 satyr ear, 221
 shell ear, 219–221
Ear surgery, 211–225
 anesthesia for, 216
 bandages after, 218
 complications, 218–219
 hospital stay for, 215–216
 medication before, 215
 myths about, 223–224
 pain and swelling after, 218
 preoperative photographs, 214
 results of, 224–225
 stitches and scars, 218

summary information, 254–255
 technique for, 217
Estrogens, prior to surgery, 49
Eyebrow lifts, 93. *See also* Forehead and brow lift
Eyelid surgery, 4, 46, 53, 89–113
 activities following, 105–106
 anesthesia for, 100–101
 bandages after, 103
 brow lifts and, 185
 bruising after, 104
 candidates for, 94–95
 complications, 108–109
 contact lenses after, 107
 hair care after, 101
 hospital stay for, 99–100
 ice compresses after, 105
 makeup after, 104–105
 medication prior to, 98–99
 pain after, 103–104
 postoperative depression, 107
 preoperative photographs, 97
 removal of stiches after, 106
 scars from, 107–108, 109
 smoking before, 99
 summary information, 254–255
 sunbathing after, 106–107, 110
 sunglasses after, 104
 tear production test prior to, 97–98
 technique for, 101–103
Eyes
 bags under, 91, 92–94, 96
 dark circles under, 94

Face peel. *See* Chemabrasion
Face-peeling parlors, 157, 162, 178. *See also* Chemabrasion; Dermabrasion
Facelifts, 39–70
 anesthetic for, 51–52
 appearing in public after, 62
 bandages, 61
 best time for, 45–46
 blood loss during, 56–57
 bruising and discoloration after, 58, 61
 chemabrasion with, 158
 complications after, 58–59
 corrections, 63
 deciding on, 40–41, 43–45

Facelifts (*cont.*)
  diagnostic tests prior to, 50
    vs. face peel, 179
  growth in popularity of, 40–41
  hair care after, 61–62
  hospital stay for, 50–52
  incisions for, 53
  makeup after, 61
  medication prior to, 48–49
  for men, 46–47, 54
  myths of, 66–68
  nerve injury from, 59–60
  numbness from, 54
  pain, 61
  postoperative depression, 62
  postsurgery procedures, 61–63
  preoperative photographs, 47–48
  "pulled look" from, 60
  recovery period, 58–59
  removal of stitches, 61
  scars, 57
  second, 66
  settling of, 63
  summary information, 254–255
  technique for, 52–54
Facial atrophy
  collagen treatment for, 207
  silicone injections for, 199, 200
Fatty cheeks, 244–245
Flap-over, for hair transplants, 223, 235–236
Food and Drug Administration
  collagen and, 209
  hair weaving and, 237
  minoxidil and, 240, 242
  silicone and, 200
Forehead
  furrow lines, 45
  wrinkles on, 158, 185, 186–187, 191
Forehead and brow lift, 42, 183–194
  alternatives to, 191
  baldness after, 187
  bandages after, 189–190
  bruising and swelling after, 190
  complications, 190–191
  hair care after, 190
  makeup after, 190
  medication before, 188–189
  pain after, 189
  preoperative photographs, 188
  preoperative procedures, 187–189

  results of, 192
  smoking before, 189
  stitches for, 190
  summary information, 254–255
  technique for, 186–187

GAX, 205
Gersuny, Dr. Robert, 197
Gillies, Sir Harold, 157
Gummy smile, correcting, 246–247

Hair, anatomy of, 229–230
Hairline
  facelift incision and, 53
  scars at, 57
Hair transplants, 227–242
  anesthesia for, 231–232
  bandages after, 238
  candidates for, 230–231
  complications, 239
  discomfort after, 238–239
  donor area for, 234
  exercise after, 239
  flap-over, 233, 235–236
  free grafts, 233–235
  medication before, 232
  postsurgical procedures, 238–239
  preoperative blood tests, 231
  preoperative photographs, 231
  results of, 237–240
  scalp preparation for, 231
  selecting doctor for, 237–238
  summary information, 254–255
  techniques for, 233–236
  strip graft, 233, 236
Hair weaving, 236–237
Hammer jaw, 78
Hands, chemabrasion on, 160
Hapsburg jaw, 78
Hematoma, 58, 63, 140
Hospital bills, 30–31
  for chin and jaw surgery, 80–81
  for ear surgery, 217
  for eyelid surgery, 101
  for facelift, 52
  for forehead and brow lift, 189
  for hair transplants, 233
  for rhinoplasty, 130–131
Hospitals, 25, 33–37
Hospital stay
  for chemabrasion, 163–164
  for dermabrasion, 173

Hospital stay (*cont.*)
    for facelifts, 50–52
    for jaw surgery, 80
Hyperpigmentation, 177
Hyperthyroidism, 96
Hypothyroidism, 96

Ibuprofen, 48
Ice compresses
    after eyelid surgery, 105
    after rhinoplasty, 134–135
Immune response, collagen and, 204

Jaw
    protruding, 78–82, 254–255
    upper, 82–84
Jaw surgery
    complications, 81–82
    summary information, 254–255
    types of, 73–74
Joseph, Dr. Jacques, 14
Juré, Dr. José, 235

Keloids
    after chemabrasion or dermabrasion, 177
    after ear surgery, 219
    after facelift, 45
    after hair transplants, 239
Keratoses, chemabrasion for, 159
Kidney disease, chemabrasion and, 163

Lasers, for facelift, 68
Lip lines, chemabrasion for, 159, 162
Lips, protruding, correction of, 246
Liver disease, chemabrasion and, 163
Long face syndrome, 84
Lop ear, 219

McCarthy, Dr. Joseph, 84
McIndoe, Sir Archibald, 9
Makeup, 12
    after chemabrasion, 168
    after eyelid surgery, 104–105
    after facelift, 61, 67–68
Manzoni, Pablo, 167
Medical insurance, 130–131

Medication
    chin surgery and, 76–78
    ear surgery and, 215
    eyelid surgery and, 98–99
    facelift and, 48–49
    forehead and brow lift and, 188–189
    hair transplants and, 232
    rhinoplasty and, 126–127
Mentoplasty. *See* Chin augmentation
Mini-lifts, 66–67
Minoxidil, 240, 242

Nasal congestion, after rhinoplasty, 136
Nasal pack, 133–134
Neck, facelift for, 42
Nerve injury, during facelift, 59–60. *See also* Numbness
Nose
    anatomy of, 121–123
    overoperated, 141
Nose surgery. *See* Rhinoplasty
Numbness. *See also* Nerve injury
    after facelift, 54
    after forehead and brow lift, 190
    after jaw surgery, 81

Open lip posture, 246–247
Orentreich, Dr. Norman, 156, 233
Orthodontia, 86
Otoplasty. *See* Ear surgery
Outpatient surgery, 35–37

Pain
    chemabrasion and, 165, 166
    chin augmentation and, 78
    ear surgery and, 218
    eyelid surgery and, 103–104
    facelift and, 60
    forehead and brow lift and, 189
    hair transplants and, 238–239
    rhinoplasty and, 134
Paraffin, liquid, 197
Passot, Dr. R., 67
Phenol, 156, 163, 164–165, 176
Postoperative depression
    after eyelid surgery, 107
    after facelift, 62
Premarin, prior to surgery, 49

INDEX

Protruding jaw, surgery for
  bandages for, 81
  hospital bill for, 80–81
  hospital stay for, 80
  numbness after, 81
  preoperative medication for, 79–80
  preoperative photographs for, 79
  summary information, 254–255
  technique, 78–82
Protruding lips, correction of, 246
"Pulled" look, from facelift, 60

Receding chin, 73
  lack of awareness of, 72
  treating, 74–78
  as "weak" chin, 86–87.
    See also Chin augmentation
Rhinoplasty, 115–152
  allegies and, 128
  anesthesia for, 129–130
  bandages for, 133–134
  bed rest and diet after, 137
  blowing nose after, 136
  candidates for, 117–120
  complications of, 140–146
  contraindications for, 123–126
  difficulty of, 121
  hair and face care after, 137
  history of, 14, 117
  limitations of, 123
  medical insurance for, 130–131
  medication before, 126–127
  myths of, 147–149
  nasal congestion after, 136
  nose injury after, 138–139
  pain after, 134
  physical activity after, 138
  preoperative photographs, 126
  preoperative precautions, 126–129
  recovery period, 135–136
  scars from, 133
  secondary procedures for, 141, 149
  smoking before, 128
  summary information, 254–255
  swelling and bruising after, 134–135, 139–140
  technique for, 131–133
  wearing eyeglasses after, 137
Rhytidectomy. *See* Facelift

Satyr ear, 221
Scars, 11
  from ear surgery, 218
  from eyelid surgery, 107–108, 109
  from facelift, 57
  of platysma muscle, 56
  from rhinoplasty, 133
Shell ears, 219–221
Silicone, 196, 198–201
Silicone injections
  for breasts, 199
  disadvantages of, 199–200
  myths about, 203–204
  procedure for, 201–202
  results of, 202–203
  summary information, 254–255
Skin
  blemishes, chemabrasion for, 159
  following chemabrasion, 168–169, 177
  elasticity, 67
  redness of, after chemabrasion or dermabrasion, 177
  sloughing, 60
  structure of, 156
  tumors, 45
  type, chemabrasion and, 159–160
Skin death, 60
Skin peeling. *See* Chemabrasion; Dermabrasion
Skin planing. *See* Dermabrasion
Skoog, Dr. Tord, 56
Smoking, surgery and, 49–50, 99, 128, 189
Spiderweb blood vessels, 159
Strip graft, for hair transplants, 233, 236
Suction lipectomy, 52–53, 54–55
  for fatty cheeks, 245
Sun protection
  eyelid surgery and, 104, 106–107, 110
  following dermabrasion, 176, 177
  importance of, 179–180
Suntanning
  cosmetic surgery and, 179–180
  eyelid surgery and, 106–107, 110
  skin wrinkles and, 154–155
Suntan parlors, safety of, 154–155

Tessier, Dr. Paul, 84

Vallis, Dr. Charles, 236
Vitamins, 48, 49
Von Graefe, Albrecht, 90

Wind, wrinkles and, 155
Witch's chin, 85
Wrinkles
  aging and, 154
  chemabrasion for, 4, 155, 158–159, 179
  complexion and, 159–160
  dermabrasion for, 179
  on earlobes, 221
  on forehead, 158, 185, 186–187, 191
  silicone treaatment for, 200–201, 202–203
  tanning and, 154–155

Zyderm II, 205, 206
Zyderm Collagen, 207
Zyplast, 207